Published by I Am Self-Publishing, 2019.

ISBN 978-1-913036-36-2

Diaries of a Sexologist's Wife

By Kerry Mars

For I.D.

Without her ideas, enthusiasm and late-night cooking in that cosy cottage kitchen, this book would not have come to be.

When you dance, your purpose is not to get to a certain place on the floor. It's to enjoy each step along the way.

Wayne Dyer

Table of Contents

The First 7 Entries

11 November, 2009

I'm writing from Sunset House, after arriving an hour early to see Evelyn. I wish she could teleport. I am so freaked out by what I discovered at Brendon's place. Yet, at the same time, I am totally in love with him.

I am about to break up with him, and that decision feels true but it also feels like a difficult thing to do. On the one hand, everything seems perfect and a dream come true.

I have not met anyone else whom I can connect with on so many levels. He is romantic, charming, charismatic, and bold. He listens so he can understand me.

BUT...

I cannot forget the LOOK he gave me. His cold treatment. His anger. His blame.

What did I do wrong?

That aside, I'm very bothered by what I saw on his computer about some secret sex club membership. He has mentioned nothing about this to me. He clearly has things to hide, and yet I somehow can't bring myself to ask!

Maybe he might surprise me. I should act cool. Already he says I'm a spoiler of fun. And since I have already somewhat decided to end things with him, it does not matter anymore, does it?

Evelyn arrives, elegant as ever in a floral bodysuit, a red tote in hand, matched with shiny red Sabrina heels. She slides her Gucci sunshades up onto her already perfectly styled straight dark hair.

"Darling, I'm soooo happy to see you!" Kerry shrieks in relief. They hug and sit down.

"What happened? You look awful."

"I want to break up with Brendon."

Evelyn curls her eyebrows up, "But you just got together with him?"

"We have a BIG GAP with sex. And I mean BIG! I'm scared. Actually, I'm TERRIFIED! He has a cupboard of whips, handcuffs, blindfolds, clamps, and he even makes his own vibrators. Well, I knew he was kind of obsessed about sex but then aren't most men?

"Then I thought, the way he's going about this is very different. I kept telling my fears to shut up. Maybe I'm just conservative and inexperienced. But the LOOK he had on his face REALLY scared me. It's like this: he started off preparing to pleasure me, and then as he took pleasure from my pleasure, he morphed, and had that silent assassin look. Well, not that I've ever seen one... OH God, I hope not!

"I mean, we've had some really rough sex, and I'd gotten really bruised. I only take it in when I shower. I mean, each time, I never fail to wonder why I allowed him to do this when I wasn't getting any true pleasure out of it... well, except to be wanted by him, to be the one who can delight him so he can enjoy himself.

"I want to please him, and I didn't want to spoil the

moment or disappoint him by telling him to stop. I loved that he took pleasure and I enjoyed the spontaneous wildness of it... but there was something not quite right, and I can't put my finger on it. I just feel I need to get out of this hole I dug and jump into, before I bury myself alive."

Evelyn did not blink. The curve of her smile went flat. "Kerry, I'm not surprised."

"What do you mean?"

"Don't get mad at me, okay?"

"I promise."

"Before you got together with him, he hit on me and tried to get in my pants. He's super seductive. My conscience never allowed me to cheat, so I've managed, just about, to stop each time. Once, when I was at his place, alone, he took me on a proper tour. In his bedroom, I made a comment about the size of his bed with all the pillars. His reply was, 'there's a lot you don't know about me.' The way he said it as his eyes seemed to search into his closet of skeletons and into me... God, I freaked out and I couldn't get out of there fast enough. So, I get what you mean about that look!"

"Why didn't you tell me?"

"I didn't want to let my experience tint your experience. Hearing you say this now, maybe I should have. Oh, I'm so sorry! I'm so glad I didn't cheat on Lex. I think if he didn't say what he said, I'd have ended up on his bed that night." Evelyn breathed out a big sigh of relief, then caught herself, "Oh my gosh, I'm so sorry, that's not how it's meant to sound."

"I'm meeting him at lunch to break up. I don't know how I'm going to do it, though. He's got his ways for reasoning and he's very, very convincing and understanding, and then I go weak. I guess I just have to be stronger." Kerry slouched, grief pulling her down.

"Yeah, you've done that once before, so you can do it again!"

"It was different then. I just blocked him out and stopped seeing him and the logic was simple. He wanted to keep the rough sex without the relationship, and it was clear cut, no need for any convincing. It was easier to say that's not for me. Now I'm a bit more invested and a bit more trapped, I guess. It was a mistake to give him airtime after two good months of peace with the silent wall I put up practically overnight!"

****

Argh, we did it again. I'm so confused. How did I get from being totally convinced I'd end it, to now, being in his flat again? I can't believe I walked in the pub and sat through watching him eat the entire lunch, unable to open my bloody mouth. But he was really adorable and understanding and such a gentleman. He wanted to know what was going on in my head, why I was thinking of breaking up, and he said I have blown my worries out of proportion. It was a slice of the pie that I did not feel good about, and he asked me to look at the rest of the pie, and how good we are for each other. *Sigh* I am such a sucker for romance. I'm so angry with myself, yet so comforted being here, and I appreciate how he's putting so much effort into allaying my worries… those bubbles and candles, and the champagne and chocolates. Oh, how I adore those puppy eyes and his warm arms around me. This time, he was super gentle, nothing like I have experienced before, and it was all soooooo romantic. I think I'm falling in love with him all over again.

11 November, 2010

Oh, my fucking God, he proposed! I thought he would never do it! I was all set to end it after this holiday. And it was far too romantic for me to say no! Now I wish I had ended the relationship before the holiday and cancelled. Then maybe I wouldn't be so confused right now. There's something not quite right about this relationship but I can't quite put a finger on it.

I should stop thinking and deal with it when I get back. He got upset when I said it was too soon to get married in May. He said he was so happy, he could get married next month. Gosh, what's happening with me? Isn't getting married what I always wanted? Heck, that was the deal breaker with Harry, and one of my niggling doubts about Brendon in the early days... this charming, bold and handsome Brendon.

Okay, let's map it out... he's intelligent and caring, and I love him. So, why am I feeling like this? Well, it didn't help that he got upset with me when I could not follow his wedding plans, which he promptly laid out almost in intricate detail soon after. He has grand plans for how he wanted the wedding to be, but I am not there yet. And I couldn't hide my shaky feelings. He was utterly disappointed that I am not as excited as he is. Oh, I feel so guilty. What the fuck is wrong with me? Why can't I just be happy? Why can't I feel the thrill? I better be careful now, because if he smells this, if I told him all this, it'd piss him off and I'm not sure anymore if I'm convinced enough to let him go. So, Kerry, be sure before you say anything more. OKAY, REMEMBER, REMEMBER!

11 November, 2011

Everything is glorious. Everything looks perfect. My best friends are all here. I'm getting married. I'm smiling but there's a part of me that is not. Even though Brendon seems to be the man of my dreams. I'm not sure why. Forget it, just smile and look freaking awesome!

11 November, 2012

He says he can't have sex with me anymore now that I'm pregnant. I'm more worried than frustrated, even though my libido is through the roof.

Pregnancy really agrees with me. I've been receiving more attention from men than I expect, for a pregnant woman. Right now, I feel relieved that he is open to us getting help. I asked if we had a problem, and his answer was yes. So, I'm on the case to find us a therapist. This woman I found looks promising. Her name is Flora. Our first session is booked and I'm counting down the days.

11 November, 2013

I have to be thankful to Flora. I don't think we would have survived this long and still be so close without her counselling sessions. But I have to say that her continuing to work with Brendon one-to-one has changed the dynamic somewhat. They've been working for months now, and I've only been in with her one-to-one twice... once on her asking and the other one, I asked to see her as I'm worried about all these tears I have been shedding for reasons I am not clear about. She wasn't able to help with that. As for the other time that I was with her, she told me to change my wardrobe and take what Brendon says as feedback instead of criticism. I questioned that, because he used to compliment my dressing up, and in fact, he still does. Anyway, I did change my wardrobe and I did buy new clothes. But either he does not like them or he paid no attention, he did not comment, and, in fact, when he noticed my new range of lingerie, he told me he felt pressured for sex and even brought it up at therapy. I feel like I cannot win.

Sex has become awkward now, sadly. I've never had sex issues with any men in the past. And of course, now I cannot make any more comparison because I am carrying our baby. That aside, I've tried to initiate, perhaps because I'm worried and looking to connect. My libido is pretty much back to normal and I can do with less sex with no big hormonal tugs... BUT I fear I may lose him. Apparently, it is rare for new mums caring for new-borns to be the first to initiate sex and I've been trying all other means to compliment him without him feeling pressured to have sex.

A relationship without sex at this stage, feels inadequate. I think if we never had a sex issue in the past, this would not worry me so much. We have spent a lot of time and money with Flora. We went to see her to address our sex issue. She brought intimacy to the table and counselled us to address that. I don't think we are very good at that, though. There's something about him that remains a mystery even if he says he tells me everything. Sitting next to him rarely feels relaxing and I feel we talk too much and too little at the same time. It's weird. That aside, we made zero progress in improving our sex situation, and we both feel unhappy about that. In fact, Brendon thinks she's out of her depth. He said that his private sessions with her had worsened his sex problems with me. That the help we are after needs to come from someone else, such as a specialist.

I don't know what to think anymore so I agreed with him. I mean, it did feel wrong when she said that if I wanted to keep Brendon and my marriage, I need to change what I wear and how groomed I look, and what I read and talk about. Despite that, I gave it a shot and put in the effort, but it seems as if it has back-fired... either that, or perhaps nothing I do will ever truly be good enough for Brendon.

On a happier note, baby Yana's arrival brought so much joy and love. My protective instinct is not unlike that of the mother cat protecting her kittens. It is a side of me that both Brendon and I have never seen before. What I am upset about is Brendon's jealousy, which simply adds to my burden. Now, I not only have to look after Yana, who clearly needs caring for, I have to consider his feelings if I don't make time for him when he comes home in the evenings. I'm not even asking him to help me out anymore because he resents that, and so if I can do the dishes and have some quiet time, or if he comes into the kitchen to hold me while I do the dishes, that would be nice.

Instead, he asks me to stop with the dishes and come to the lounge and relax with him, but I can't relax for more than ten minutes without feeling the pull of the dishes, because at the back of my mind, I know the baby could wake up any minute and I feel sleepy already and I'd hate to wake up in the morning with a sink full of dishes, a screaming baby, and no baby utensils. More importantly, it was how he said what he said, after two hours of listening to him at dinnertime. "How are you prioritising? You had the whole day to do the chores, but you chose the time when I came home to do it, instead of spending time and relaxing together."

And no, it is not that he wants sex, so he is definitely not angry that I was not available to him for sex, but he is not recognising my predicament as the primary carer. In fact, I sense jealousy and resentment from him now that the baby has arrived.

11 November, 2014

sigh I don't remember when I have ever felt so sexual and sexy and undesired by my partner all at the same time. We just finished the first bundle of sex coaching with someone Brendon found.

I had my reservations when he brought this to the table. I felt that what's happening between us is more than just sex, and sex is the symptom. Anyhow, I'm glad I parked that aside long enough to see this through. Madame Butterfly got us talking about sex and it was very intimately educational to say the least. It made the topic safe somewhat easier to discuss. If anything at all, I have a clearer picture of this 'big sex GAP' between Brendon and I, that I intuitively felt but never truly understood. If not for the so-called GAP, I may not have learnt all this, as I never had any problems with sex with anyone else before Brendon, but I was also probably more clueless.

I am embarrassed that I did not know many terms and phrases that were used in the room. I feel insulted by Brendon when he rolled his eyes, but most of all, that he did not share resources or educational material on sex with me, but 'shared' far too much that was more a put-down instead of an uplift or to empower me with knowledge.

I don't blame him. I mean, it would be a threat if I grew more confident in my own sexuality while he is insecure about his own sexuality, wouldn't it? And knowing how he drew satisfaction in putting people back to their own places, he probably derived some satisfaction from being the one more plugged into the scene.

The big gift from our sessions with Madame Butterfly is the point she made about not making the guy the centre of my universe. She also added that the more I did that, the more Brendon would feel suffocated, and the only reference point I could control is my own. There is no way I can use his behaviours or responses as an indication of my own growth.

This was BIG for me, because it was counterintuitive. It seemed logical and natural to assume that improvements in the feedback and criticism from Brendon meant I was doing something right, and anything contrary meant I was not hitting the mark. I took things too personally, so when Madame Butterfly suggested that I learn to ignore his feedback and behaviours, not take his words too seriously since he was constantly shape-shifting, and instead, focus on improving what I set out to improve for myself and for the marriage, I struggled with the concept but welcomed the freedom, even though I felt quite lost...

Her words still ring clearly… "you need to be able to swing with the punches and not internalise everything too much as he's ever-changing," and "you need to own your own evolution in clarity and strength, with clear boundaries yet remaining open and flexible."

"Swing with the punches." Madame Butterfly, thank you, you do know.

She told me to read up on David Deida's work, and so far, I have enjoyed learning from this man. I feel my armour melting away, slowly but surely, and as I feel less and less fear, ironically, I feel myself growing into the character played by Cate Blanchett in Elizabeth, when she rode that white horse. Hmmm... I like the image that just came to mind.

What I also struggled with was 'praise.' I never thought he needed praise, to be honest. When Madame Butterfly suggested that I decide what I wanted Brendon to do and praised him whenever he inched closer towards what I wanted, I got goose-bumps faster than an allergic reaction. My first reaction was that it was patronising, like I'm some kind of mistress talking to a pet dog. Then my gut wrenched in rebellion, "I'm not raising a son, damn it! I want a man, not a boy!"

But you know what... I married him and I want a happy marriage. I don't want to lose him. And if he needs help knowing what he did that pleases me, and if praise is the only way he can hear me, then praise I will, even if it does give me goose bumps!

Another thing I am still finding it hard to do is to state what I want and then feeling completely ignored, dismissed, or worse, disrespected and trampled on. I would rather not say what I want from him and avoid those painful feelings.

On a lighter note, I'm laughing now, as I remember cringing when Madame Butterfly advised me to slow my movements right down, slow my speech right down, and dance everyday by spiralling my hips in an infinity symbol. I have to say, this particular 'homework' had me in stitches as I caught a glimpse in the mirror at how ridiculous I looked. I look like a clunky, chunky, clumsy, cow! My God! First, I have a constantly noisy baby around me, a mind full of tasks and planning ahead, a baby routine that helps me but dictates my day pretty much... to slot in dance? That is a 'bit' of a JOKE.

But I wrote to Madame Butterfly, because I was cracking my head about how to, in her words, "grow my man" while also growing my femininity. And then her words touched me and broke me at the same time. I just cried, perhaps simply from exhaustion.

"You are amazing and beautiful. You can figure this out and what will work. Treat every day as a laboratory and do your experiments. It is fun. It's actually a very fascinating subject.

"You may wish to imagine you are some courtesan who is playing at seducing the emperor to bring out your playfulness. Brendon is a guy who gets bored easily... if you had to fight off other competitors in the palace, wouldn't you work really hard at it by being creative?"

Since our last session with Madame Butterfly, Brendon has been deep into his mood swings again. Our last session ended with him challenging her in an angry tone, "You seem to be taking her (as in my) side. I think it's because you're taking the female perspective. You don't know the male perspective."

Today, his mood lifted a little, as he toyed with the idea of getting the same qualification as her, to become the male counterpart, if you may. I joked that, "You don't need a doctorate to solve our intimacy problems, do you?" and we both laughed.

That's what I like about us. We can do the serious talk

shit, and the fact that he is into personal growth continues to give me hope. But it leaves me feeling like I'm running on a hamster wheel, like there's a dangling bait in front of me that promises light at the end of the tunnel, except I can never reach the end of the tunnel.

BUT, I am noticing my discomfort with the idea of him operating as a sexologist, and this is unravelling bit by bit, in layers. What this means for our day-to-day routine and our marriage I don't know. All I can do is support his decision.

11 November, 2015

Wow, where has the year gone? So much has happened. I have been busy fire-fighting this turmoil. It seemed like only yesterday that Brendon began the programme. Soon, he will be graduating. Reading my last entry made me realise how differently I feel today, about sexuality, about me as a woman, and about my marriage.

From where I stand today, I can feel the difference between how I am today versus 'back then'... how I was so totally clueless about sexuality as a subject, and where I stood in regards to my opinion and belief system, yet completely oblivious about my lack of knowledge and understanding.

I remember vividly sending Brendon off for his first training module. The excitement in his eyes matched the degree of hopefulness I held onto in my heart. I thought to myself, "Perhaps this will bring him happiness. Perhaps he'll find his answers. Perhaps this will give him a sense of meaning and lift his depression. Perhaps this will bring us closer, bring passion and intimacy into our marriage. Perhaps, perhaps."

I remember the devastation that followed when Brendon returned full of expectations of my being able to answer his questions, being able to meet his latest discoveries and lessons. I remember feeling my heart crumble bit by bit as I tried to buffer the pain of humiliation and embarrassment, sitting right next to an intently listening older couple at a local coffee shop, trying to prove to him that nothing he said or did would bother me. I was trying to prove that I am more spiritual and less egotistical than he was, that I was this bigger, greater person who took the high road. Clearly, I failed and miserably so.

Brendon had begun to "talk down" at me angrily at the coffee shop, asking me sex-related questions while the old couple who sat next to us listened to everything. He expected me to have all the answers to his questions and he got all worked up as I struggled to comprehend the conversation, let alone find my words. It was like one terrible nightmare of an interrogation. Eventually, I got snappy, and that left me feeling rotten by nightfall. How ridiculous, I thought, that from one day to the next, he expected me to be as 'knowledgeable' as him about the subject?!

What is he thinking…? It's bad enough that I did not know half the terms he was using at the sessions with Madame Butterfly; I wished he was kind and brave enough to talk to me all this while. Perhaps things would have turned out differently. It was as if he chose her in order to fix me and with that, to fix our intimacy problems. Thanks to her matter-of-factness, and our separate one-time, individual sessions, and all the resources she pointed out to me, I found the space to truly tune into my inner voice. If not for her encouragement to focus on strengthening myself, I don't think my anger would surface to balance my fear of upsetting him or fear of losing him.

I am glad I went with him to his graduation party. I got a sense for the kind of colleagues he would have in this field. These experiences help me grow in my capacity to be radically inclusive, to open my mind and see the beliefs I never knew I held in my system, in order to shape them up according to how I choose to believe from thereon.

I never really developed any sophistication in terms of language to talk about sex. I didn't even know what BDSM stood for, let alone the intricacies of each dimension in that umbrella term. I did not even know that what I enjoyed was called Vanilla sex, and that this wasn't necessarily the norm; it was the least shunned upon and therefore more widely discussed and accepted. I never knew that mutually consenting and respectful Polyamorous relationships and open marriages even existed.

I learnt that no one has any real control or say over what arouses them, and libido is just as unique; we all have our own distinct sexual fingerprint. And since I came to know this truth, I developed a newfound compassion for individuals who found themselves aroused by subjects and objects that societies or local communities had deemed inappropriate. Never in a million years would I have considered sex workers, sex therapists, or sex business owners to be part of my network.

Thanks to Brendon, I spent a whole summer reading sex books... And as my mind opened, my experience of life began to shift.

Yes, it was VERY difficult to have the conversations we have had in regards to our Open Relationship/Marriage. Yes, I got convinced in the summer months to give it a go. In fact, I found myself surprisingly excited because just as I said yes to Brendon, I met Nate. He was handsome and something sparked from the moment our eyes locked. Meeting Nate led me to some of the most life-changing experiences, and the most important lesson of all, was the understanding that sexual energy is a highly potent force of creation.

The desire to be filled completely by a man, with a body to-die-for, a gaze to-pour-out-for, a touch to-melt-into, was powerful, and for the first time in my life, I allowed myself to feel that desire, overwhelming as it was, and shameful as it was to me back then: "No 'good girl' enjoys sex. A 'good girl' reserves her vagina and opens her legs only to the one man she loves. If you enjoy sex, you're a tramp." The list goes on.

I never slept with Nate in the end. He got into a committed relationship before any deeper discussions or agreement was reached, so nothing happened between us. Meeting him was like a Divine arrangement…the timing was impeccable and the angel signs were everywhere. Our conversations allowed me to begin the journey of separating between lust, romance, limerence and love.

The game changer was that Nate introduced me to a whole new dimension of spirituality. I made new friends in his close-knit 'golden' circle, each member totally accepting of me in all my bruises from self-hatred. Nate was my angel in disguise. He was an angel that held me with light hands and wings and the energy led me towards an externalised teacher, in the form of a former hermit spirit guide, grandparents plant medicine, and groups of soul sisters.

As he and his spiritual family went to Burning Man, I made my way to a remote village to study energy. I had so many profound experiences dancing while lying down on a mat, surrounded by pure vibrations of nature and sound, taking no drugs or any sort of sacred medicine. I was awake in a dream-like state, able to move yet feeling paralysed at the same time, in total surrender while having all sorts of visions and shared visions, all of which continues to teach me so much about how connected we all are.

There was one hilarious moment. I awoke from one of the energy dance experiences, hearing my inner self go, "Oh my God, how am I going to share what just happened to me? This is SO EMBARRASSING!" And when, one by one, people started to share, I heard my inner self go, "Oh my God, I'm NOT ALONE!"

It's so crazy. I had a vision of a fire-blowing dragon entering my vagina and coming out from my mouth, then coiling around me as if making love, then twirling around my neck before kissing me and going into me again, lifting my chest really high, before coming out of my vagina as if it was being birthed right in that moment. So, when a guy shared this same vision, and he has no vagina to begin with, all my fears melted away. I simply relaxed and laughed and the room felt like One.

The more raw food I ate, the more my body and her channels opened up. The more 'weird' people like me who I met, the more normal I seemed to myself, and the more people opened up to me. My whole being just kept expanding.

Everyone is coping with life, so who am I to judge how they ought to be coping? How can I say that being gender-fluid is wrong when I do not know what it feels like on a day-to-day basis? Who is to say that continuing to expand our relationship instead of breaking up is morally superior because it demonstrates our tremendous capacity for great love... nor the contrary, that the mature way is to face a break-up even though it is hard to do.

Sexuality and spirituality, labels aside, feels the same. There is a oneness and a pleasure that is personal and hard to describe. There is the chase and the elusiveness from the seeking of it. And there is the letting go aspect necessary in order to fully get into the experience. There's a fine line between creating happy boundaries versus not 'needing' them as the ego continues to dissolve... as it does with both sexual and spiritual evolution.

Wow Kerry, look at what you have learnt! I really ought to write a book!

*****

The Kink Conference was quite something. It was a strange experience, to dress sexy, but to not feel sexy at all. It was eye-opening to bear witness to the broad range of what is defined by this group of people as 'kink.'

I was comforted and enjoyed being with Brendon, walking through the cubicles, holding hands, even though it was not my thing. Even so, I loved being able to peek into his world, and to see people have fun playing, with what constitutes 'adult privileges.'

After the conference, what I enjoyed most of all was our conversation over tapas about how it was for us... I loved sharing that experience, that moment, and somehow, our little private huddle over those tiny mysterious bite-sized parcels was more intimate and sexual than the kink weekend.

BUT... what I did not share in full depth with Brendon was the 'aha' moment I had when I met a completely monogamous couple, who renewed their intimacy with kink, now that their children have grown up. I longed for the kind of intimacy that couple embodied. I guess it showed me the bruised side of my heart after Brendon suggested having an open relationship and marriage in order for him to find other play partners since he knew BDSM was not my thing. He said I was inauthentic, and doing it just to get close to him, when I should be focusing on finding my own sexual identity, and meeting him on par.

I'm afraid I am much less interested in sex as a subject to debate about, compared to him. I'm happy to follow his lead, but it seems as if following his lead does not cut it. I remember when we first started dating, he wanted to do funny stuff with me, playing with my vagina and watching how he could make it squirt. After a number of hours being in the bubble tub with him, I was not enjoying myself anymore, and he got very upset when I said in my most gentle voice, with some hesitation and trepidation, 'Please stop, I'm not enjoying this anymore.' I expected him to at least say 'okay' or kiss me. However, he threw his hands up, splashing water everywhere, and stormed off. Then at dinner, he sulked the entire time and eventually murmured that I was too uptight. As this occurred early on in the relationship, I merely concluded, 'How rude!' But the underlying beliefs that generated that reaction haven't changed much.

Recently, he started to pursue Amani, our neighbour. Can you believe that? I was obviously upset because I see that bitch every day. What he doesn't know is that we talk. All women talk.

When I finally agreed to an open marriage, it was under

the context of him wanting to develop his sexual being into fullness. It was part of his personal development, and I said yes, because I just want him to be happy. I believe we can develop in many ways, but to say no to him to pursue his desires felt like I would have been setting rules, which I had zero control over. And at the end of the day, why would anyone want to do that? Why would anyone want to control someone they love, if ultimately, we want to see our loved ones happy?

Ideally, I want him to be devoted to me. To want to play with me, with care and respect. To bring me along on his journey. To teach me. To guide me. To share experiences. To talk about our days. To be "normal," whatever that means.

We had a heated argument at cocktails one evening, before our rough sex date in town. He told me to wait for him at a fairly classy hotel basement bar, but it was known to be a hooker bar. I didn't realise until I was there and had 'hungry' men looking at me. I kept moving about so no one could come near me, and it was then that I overheard a negotiation taking place and I finally realised it was a hooker bar. I made my way to the toilet and messaged Brendon to come soon or move me to the next location.

What was supposed to be a night of kinky play turned into a consented spanking, where I took the beatings. I was keen to try it for some twisted spiritual reasons. I would love to be able to transcend the human bodily pain to get into the pleasure realm, the sub space, and meet him there, from a state of spiritual transcendence.

Having been through an extended hypnobirthing before, I thought this would be the perfect ground to expand myself. In hindsight, I realise that I must have craved intimacy with him so much, and I must have craved being desired by him so much, I would do anything to make our sex problems go away. I broke down by the end of it. I don't think it was the physical pain as such, even though the aftermath was numbing. My cry felt like it came from hurt residing deep within. I remember blanking out and I caught myself thinking, why am I doing this when it is not what I want, but it is a workaround to get what I want, which is intimacy with my husband?

Anyway, I was very upset that he wanted to convert Amani into his lifestyle. He said that her husband did not have to know. I disagreed. An open relationship is not a free for all. An open relationship is just that, OPEN. The whole point of it was to have No Deception. The minute there is deception, it is no longer open. You see, I never would have been able to argue this and be so comfortable standing in my own Light of Truth, so to speak, if not for my lessons with one of his faculty. I'm lucky to have that teacher reachable at the touch of a button, supporting me on this 'lifestyle,' coaching me from his years of experience.

Where are Brendon's bloody ethics? He is not walking what he preaches. I said to him that I am supportive of the work he is doing, I believe he is helping people to heal shame and guilt around sex, and I am proud of some of his messages... BUT, if he continues seeing Amani with full awareness of what he is doing and keeping her and her husband in the dark space of deceit, he is crossing ethical boundaries. And I can no longer be proud of him professionally. And I can no longer be silenced by his disrespect.

I think he heard me, because one evening he came back looking rather despondent and said that Amani had told him her husband would never agree to that. Ah, I thought, he acted on my feedback and had that conversation with her. Yet, he was still seducing her, texting her from our bed one night, and he told me off for asking him why he was doing that when he agreed he wasn't going to play with her anymore.

I had a meltdown. It was one of those nights where I cried until I hyperventilated and my leg cramped up. I called for him to help me get out of the mess of snot and tears. He eventually threw a towel on me. I felt something snap in my heart that night. My inner voice resolved and I vowed never to allow myself to get into that state again.

In the weeks after those two crying spells, I noticed not much had changed in the dynamic between us, as a couple, and in our sex life. The more focus we put on trying to solve it, the more it seems it is becoming unwieldy... or shall I say, the more we are pulling apart rather than coming together. I don't think it's about not enough effort on our individual parts... it feels more like a manifestation of our dynamic in the bedroom that is the challenge, and we are trying to resolve it by going technical.

*****

Hmm... after all that venting, now I can't sleep. I have been mulling over everything. I am suffering. I see the pattern I am in. I seek validation from Brendon and put his needs ahead of mine, believing they are mine too. It is my default and constant, which makes it unhealthy and imbalanced. Then I struggle with the aftermath.

I first explored BDSM in an uneducated way as I wanted to be chosen by him as someone to be exclusive with. I then married him because of everything we have shared.

I notice that while I have reasons to agree with sexual exploration, the underlying reason is that I just want to be with him, and this is how I am showing him that I love him. It is confusing because it seems like that's what I want, but this sort of want does not arise within me naturally on its own. So, after a while, I get to a point where for one reason or another, my truth wants to be heard, and I have not been very good at listening to it because my insecurities are ruling my actions and I am afraid of expressing discomfort because I find it hard to find the words. Plus, often words are extremely limiting and easily misunderstood, and I know it pisses him off, so I try to wait for the right words to come before I can open my mouth. Hmm... the word abandoned just came to me. Perhaps, I had abandoned myself here.

Wow... anyway, I wrote to tell him what's going on with me.

Hello darling,

2015 has been a hell of a year for me. Emotionally, it's been a big roller coaster even if I don't appear as stormy on the surface. I feel a sense of completeness although this doesn't really make sense considering we seem to still be journeying based on what we agreed.

I have come to terms with our relationship. I will not hold on to any hopes or ideals for they take me away from the present-day gifts of our partnership. I will not seek sexual fulfilment outside our partnership for it takes away the invisible opportunity for me to heal what needs to be healed right here right now.

It is almost synchronous that I felt readier than ever to take my work to the next level. I feel held again and in my space, ready to engage.

I love you and I take you as you are. I do need a little help from time to time with this as we keep evolving. The help I need is to be affirmed by emotional intimacy and physical contact.

My intention is to make choices that ultimately feel good deep within, from a place of safety... choosing to create with awareness and understanding of consequences, choosing to create by walking the path that values life and serves my whole system in health; in love and freedom.

Look forward to our next big chat. I'd better go sleep now.

Kxx

We never had the next big chat, the way I envisaged it... I felt pushed by his anger and in that moment, I blurted out, "I don't want an open relationship."

It isn't something I want or need at this time. It scatters my energy too much.

11 months Trilogy (I)

11 January, 2016

Two months have gone by. I don't know how I am truly feeling. The holiday with his family went okay, but I was comfort eating a lot... I also laughed in groups and cried in private, loads, like I was in a washing machine. I'm not sure if any of his family and friends noticed the turmoil going on in my marriage. We put up a very united front, very loving and understanding and supportive.

Brendon speaks of me proudly. He is proud of us and sings praises about how good we are as a couple, and how we only have sophisticated problems and sophisticated ways to deal with them.

I agree with him to some extent... the challenge is indeed different, but I'm not convinced it is easier! I wrote to him...

Darling,

This past week has been difficult for me. I have been grieving a lot and I feel lonely in my effort to sort out our relationship and marriage. It is as if we are finally returning to address our relationship challenges after a detour (assuming divorce or a slow painful death of connection leading to divorce is not our chosen option).

You had said before that our sexual challenge is where our relationship difficulty unfortunately is expressing itself. I do agree with you. I feel much less trusting than before, almost like a betrayal, as a result of this thing with Amani. It feels different from jealousy. With jealousy I would clock envy. I do not envy her and neither do I feel that I am less than her. In this scenario, I have experienced defensiveness and attack, and felt disrespected. It will take me awhile to get my gear back and I need your patience and reassurance, not in the form of reporting (I hate this myself) but in the form of avoiding behaviours that trigger me, like being elusive/hiding stuff. I do not like this feeling I am carrying of being afraid to ask you specific things about your day because I do not want to trigger you either. This combination, I feel, is driving our hearts further away from each other, not closer.

Our journey in 2015 has brought me great experiences. It has brought me back to me, a higher version of me, and I am forever grateful to you for all your support. I have no doubt about your love for me, and I have no doubt about my love for you, even if we are still learning how to communicate our love such that the other feels it. I know we hold a similar vision but what we want may not be the same things at the same time, and this is the challenge.

I know you are upset about my choice to not have an open relationship. I do not know whether you will honour my choice because even though I heard you say that you value our relationship a lot, you are clear about what you want in terms of having play partners. I can understand why this might be fun to do and almost perhaps a dream come true, and I am truly sorry that I am unable to do this for you. I think that when there is a specific event that may lead to sexual activity, I can consent, for example, Burning Man or Dungeon visits. But I do not wish to have other relationships coexisting in our marriage, especially at this time when we have a young family, which I'm hoping to grow. I'd love to have more family time and to be able to enjoy that together, and I need all my resources for that. At the same time, I want to be grateful that we still have each other to explore our sexuality with each other, instead of wishing for something else. In my journey, I had learned that it was because of my baggage with you that I might not have considered you as a fun and willing partner for sacred spiritual practices, but today, I feel deep joy that I can share this with you, even if you eventually still choose not to.

But if you do feel that what we have at this time (our marriage, our relationship, our partnership, our family, and our exclusivity) is not what you want and you are compromising a core identity of yours (leather and whips with many partners), then we need to discuss. I am also curious to understand why my openness to try new things, things that you may do with your partner, does not make me a play partner, and how are we each responsible for creating that, and what we will do for our part?

Letting our egos and our shadows continue to rule will only drive us further apart. Then we won't just have little sex, we will have nothing left but a history.

I love us, not for the memories we have created together, but for what we are choosing to create on a daily basis, and the more we can get to a constructive, grateful, joyful place regularly, the more likely we are to grow our happiness. And isn't happiness ultimately what we are seeking?

At some point, I'd love for us to bring to surface the hidden rules we are currently operating by, and may have never discussed, so we can look at them and decide if some of these inherited rules are what we want to carry forward. I think this exercise will help me tremendously.

I know that I am still hurting, and just now was an example... When I said, I'm writing a love letter and you said to whom, and then you said you never know these days... I retorted, "I know" with anger. I am holding the anger because I am unhappy about what has happened and we don't have an agreement. Holding this anger inside me is not serving us even though I think it is mine to deal with. See what I mean by how easily we can start divorcing emotionally?

I am free on Tuesday if you are. We can sit down again to discuss.

Much love.

So much has been happening and now I find myself yet again sitting with raw, vulnerable, sad, hopeful, calm, anxious feelings all at the same time. The past weeks have been difficult.

For months I had been hiding my truth... that I did not want to have an open relationship, and when I finally had the courage to say it, I am going through the pains of that revelation, perhaps for which I had known and feared and therefore tried to avoid.

The year 2015 was filled with dilemmas and gifts of experience, mostly because I followed Brendon into them, pushing my boundaries. In July, we agreed to have an open relationship and that brought its own challenges and gifts, but we were in it together. After some exploration, and during this time nothing sexually had taken place with any other person for Brendon and I, as far as I'm aware, I am back to square one feeling like a different person.

I felt differently about monogamy in that it became a

more conscious choice and I did not feel a need to explore my sexuality with other people and have other romantic or sexual relationships alongside my marriage. I also have a vision of a family life and I want to be fully resourced to enjoy that. However, I did not want to impose my decision on Brendon since I had already agreed, so I sat on it for two months. Until I had the courage to let go of the marriage that I had been trying hard to keep and trusting that little Yana will be fine. It is so hard to be authentic in the midst of fear and grief. It is even harder to work on letting go of my ego while trying to grow self-respect and set boundaries.

Now I am going through similar pains to infidelity, almost like a punishment. Brendon has withdrawn emotionally and I have grieved loads. He says he is not ready to discuss this further and he wants to remain married for now. I feel his anger and pain despite his coldness and I am wondering what my best course of action is–to leave or to stay like this.

When I break down in front of him, there's a part of me that wants him to know yet I feel worse because I feel so pathetic when his reaction is apathy. If I rule out leaving him, I feel pain, I feel victimised, and that my boundaries will not be respected. But leaving seems to suggest that I am the one manifesting the separation, which is not what I want.

*****

I feel like I am sitting on a thin wall of hope, staring at the green fields in front of me, but noticing this deep and dark abyss beneath me that is paralysing me in fear.

Last night, after a good dose of dancing and laughter

and drinks with the girls, I walked home with my face streaming with tears, and I heard myself. I have lost intimacy with him, and this is the key to many problems. I long for intimacy and did what I could to get it, but the more I do that, the more I chased it away.

It is not easy not to feel anything, whether I decide to stay or leave. It seems as if both are difficult but leaving feels like it will change the direction of my energy. I am starting to see the deeply embedded beliefs I held about family and relationship, about marriage, and about sex.

F*g beliefs!

Clearly it was doing its thing. I wonder – am I afraid of freedom or am I unable to feel freedom?

It is strange to feel this. I have been with men who are control-oriented and fear-based, who held me tightly wrapped in so much need and shallow stability. Yet, in my current situation, I don't feel free.

I know that many men and women philander, with bodies and minds – it's all part of being human. I have learnt to hold myself with elegance and grace, like a queen, holding the belief that sex is but one part of the human experience, and at the end of the day, the king always returns to his palace.

Brendon and I are both clearly feeling pain in all this, whether it is because of guilt, anger, grief or hidden shame it doesn't really matter. I cannot control my feelings when they arise, but I can take responsibility for what to do based on my situation. This is the only way out of this pain.

Right now, I am not ready to walk out.

Darling,

I am filled with a deep sadness about us, and where we are at today. But I feel immense gratitude and joy as well, for all that we have shared. It is not easy to remember everything without hoping that we will continue to build a life together in such a balanced, harmonious, fulfilling and memorable way. Equally, letting go of that hope is not easy.

Our dynamics have changed and I'm certain you feel this too. It has been changing, but the shift is clearer and I think this is because I have drawn a boundary. The distance between us sometimes feel wider than the ocean even though we are cordial and courteous, and my heart remains where it has always been: devoted to you.

I feel different these days whenever I try to speak freely with you, and while I cannot be fully certain why, I suspect it is because I sense your protective wall or resistance that is closing off the anger which needs to be processed… all of which I sincerely respect and understand.

My growth challenge has been about trusting that my heart is safe with you; from the moment we got together I fully trusted you with my heart. This can, at times, be particularly scary and when I am scared, my anxiety escapes to test whether I have done the right thing.

On my part, I am now wondering what all that has transpired in 2015 culminating in that fateful conversation last month means for us from this point on.

And when I think about this, I find myself asking what my best next steps are... to continue living like this until something else happens, or consider what alternatives I really have and can they be explored or discussed or otherwise...? And what these would practically mean for us on a day-to-day basis?

I feel nervous about the myriad of possibilities that can unfold with a single decision. Equally I am curious because they are unknown and by that definition, it will be an adventure that I am delighted and privileged to embark on.

This is where I'm at today. I'm ready to catch up on this whenever you are (not because I have processed everything and need to talk, but to keep connected in the processing, which I believe is the key to any healthy relationship... there can be no real relationship without honest connection).

Take all the time you need and I will do the same. I hold the intention to be as honest as I can be, as we enter the next stage, all in perfect timing. And as I hear you enter the deep snooze, I wish you a beautiful morning and weekend.

Brendon replied saying that he chooses to remain married. That he hasn't ruled out sexual exploration but is happy to park it for now, and he reminded me that little Yana and I remain his priority.

It was a very sweet message in that it seems to be saying all the right things. Yet, the human experience of him is quite different. He has been rather cold. And no, we haven't had any make-up sex, let alone any deep or meaningful kisses nor conversations.

It is a rough time, and I noticed that my anger is coming out in ways that are unrefined for a lady. The other day, I felt this enormous build-up of energy in my belly and heart that wanted to scream out at him. I hated his look and how he dismisses me by ignoring me totally, like I don't exist. How did I allow this to reach this stage? All those times of counselling are simply pointless. They are like band aids to a horrible marriage of two people who are so unhappy.

Next week we will be experiencing sexual healing based on native American and Tao traditions from two Shamans. I don't feel up for it, obviously, because our situation today is vastly different from when we booked it. Maybe we need it more on a personal level now than professionally.

Anyhow, united front it shall be. We will be hosting friends and friends of friends to meet with these two Shamans.

11 February, 2016

OMG!

The time with the Shamanic Queens was soooooo worth it!

I never imagined it to be this good! I never thought we would be able to make this leap!

I am over the moon!

It is indeed true that with intimacy, one can feel quite literally, invincible!

This was how it went:

The prep work was all about feeling into the current situation, then physically, we were given exercises to de-armour, which essentially is about freeing up space through touch, what we hold onto in our bodies with regards to sexual beliefs... to remove shame and guilt and to send love and open the space up for new memories to come into the body.

Then, on the third day, I got a call early in the morning to bring sexy clothes along. Brendon was told to leave the room for 30 minutes while I was briefed. I would be playing the Tao Tigress. When I received the instructions, I did my best to keep a straight face, while my mind conjured up the images of what would come... and I looked, in my mind, like a blend of the sex worker and the concubine. I was laughing inside – a nervous laugh filled with doubt as to whether I could pull this off!

And guess what?

I DID IT!!!!

It was awesome. I had never felt so sexy and powerful, dominant and submissive, all at the same time! I am incredibly happy to be able to pleasure Brendon! I never thought I could pleasure him. If anything, perhaps this showed him that BDSM is not the only way he can find pleasure.

You know what he said?

That this is the sexiest he has ever seen me be.

The trick – my domination is in leading the energy, my submission comes through via the physical positioning and stance. It worked like magic!

I guess the entire set up helped. The best part was that Brendon shared one of the most intimate workings of his mind in a long time, and the shift in his energy is observable, as if he grew from a spoiled brat of a boy to a powerful man surrendering to this seductress he felt safe with. It's incredible!

By the end of the day, I felt as if we could conquer anything. My conclusion is that when a couple can truly connect in a deep way through sex and intimacy, nothing can 'break' their union.

11 March, 2016

Sadly, the honeymoon effect from training with the Shamanic Queens is wearing off. I feel that we are struggling to come up to speed. It is becoming awkward. I still have Skype calls with Shamanic Queens, and from their feedback, and how vital I feel and look, I must be doing something right.

Then why are we like this again in the bedroom! It's so frustrating!

Brendon says he is feeling pressured again. I have no idea why. I don't feel that I am overconfident, nor do I put any pressure on him to perform. The way he is describing it, it feels a lot like someone dealing with insomnia... the anticipation and perception of expectations creates the anxiety perhaps?

Or maybe it is getting repetitive and boring... But if it is, then just bloody say it and we can do something about it.

sigh I have no clue.

11 April, 2016

The gap between us is getting bigger. This time, I am truly afraid. He is not talking to me anymore, and I have nothing to say to him that is interesting, apart from snippets from the day that I remember about our baby's life... and she isn't much of a baby anymore.

He shares absolutely nothing about his work, whereas he used to spend a couple of hours every night talking about his day. He would wait for me to finish with my bedtime routine and come out to watch a movie over tea. These days, he is catching up with his research and if we watch anything, it involves sex education in one form or another. Once, we had friends over to watch Nymphomania. When they left, he snapped at me, saying that I was competing with him at the post-movie discussion. Things have vastly changed. When we both used to work in the same field, he had greater respect for me and my opinion. Now he either says I'm competing with him or I don't know what I'm talking about... not just verbatim, but through every pore of his being. Well, he is the one who is qualified now anyway, so perhaps yes, he is indeed the educated one. But I don't think it is a license for him to speak to me like that. Maybe he is resentful, maybe he is stressed, maybe he is angry. In any case, I cannot live like this... simply looking like a yummy mummy who got it together, while walking on eggshells, keeping my mouth shut, particularly if I have a different opinion from him in his area of 'expertise,' like sexology.

11 May, 2016

I hate myself. I am so angry with myself. I am upset that I did not firmly uphold my decision to not attend his event with Yana and sitter. I should have followed my instincts. This is clearly not the first time, so what else will it take for me to be clear about what I would do as a mother of Yana, not a mother of Brendon?

Brendon wanted me to attend all his open events, the first run of six he had put up, to market his services. I attended the first because I could come after Yana was asleep. But for the second one, he asked me to go earlier, so I had to bring Yana along, which was also what he wanted. I sat through his session, trying to be as supportive as I could be, with Yana wailing downstairs with the sitter the entire time. Eventually, she came up to the room, and as she sat with me, I realised that the topic was unsuitable for her age, so I left the room with her. It was as if we were props, there for show, totally out of place, yet Brendon was glad we went and still expected us to attend the next one. I knew there and then that will be the last open event we will attend altogether for a while.

11 June, 2016

Since Brendon went public with his new persona, I have been asked by mutual friends what brought on the change, and how we were. For many, we exemplify the role model couple, the one functioning at the leading edge. But as I read his blogs and responded to the questions, I felt like I was living a lie.

Brendon would ask for my opinion, and quite often, I would find his articles well-researched and sometimes well-written. BUT, many times I felt a gut reaction and cringed– times when I felt it did not sound like him at all. Perhaps it is normal, to know more, being behind the scenes. However, there is a distinction in that I am unable to give him my honest opinion anymore. I used to, and to my horror, he said, "I don't want to know your opinion, I just want to know if it reads well." From then on, another part of me died.

11 July, 2016

Visiting my parents at this difficult time of my life is bringing me such a relief. I obviously never shared the details of my marital struggles with them, and what they know is the facade of it. Well, to be fair, Brendon and I do get along well when we are with others... well, actually, I take back my words. Once, he planned a surprise by somewhat hijacking the family birthday party I had planned jointly to celebrate with my dear brother, and then he got really upset with me when it did not go to plan. Obviously, because I had no idea about the surprise, I showed up at the venue before he did! I was concerned about Yana being hungry and us being late for the table reservation, and because he was late, I thought I'd go up and get Yana sorted out first. To my surprise, I saw my friends there, and they all said, "Surprise!" I was indeed surprised, but when Brendon came up, his face was black like the Chinese Wok! He angrily passed me my birthday card while saying, "Here, you just had to spoil it," and then he stormed off. Apparently, he was upset because he did not get to see my surprised look. I didn't spoil my birthday. He did. I decided to have fun with my friends nonetheless. But it was different after that "ceremonious" start.

11 August, 2016

This is the month when it all happened. The birth, the death, the rebirth. Crazy. It is the month we celebrate our wedding anniversary, and the month I know I have to get out of this prison. I am keeping myself there for far too long. Yes, largely it is my perception, and I have felt free while living together. BUT, true freedom comes from being able to really honour my body, my mind, my heart, my spirit... my whole.

That night shall be the last conversation we will have as a couple about our future. I have never felt so bullied and trapped. So inauthentic and silenced. Unimportant, lonely and unloved. He could still smirk, while I felt totally crushed inside. With what he said, he could have equally yielded his whip and bat on my body, then the damage would have been more visible.

He has the potential to kill, that I know, but he also has great restraint, so it's got to come out somehow, somewhere... through his vibe, through his words, through his behaviours. He is protective too, of course, perhaps over-protective, particularly regarding how others treat Yana and I, but that's not the point. The point is that he is killing me softly with his song.

How do I get out of this?

A million things crossed my mind in those wee hours of the morning. I know I cannot handle him. I can only see how things will escalate very quickly and go out of control. I need to find a way out of this asap. Gosh, I feel like I am hatching a plan to escape from my captor! Perhaps I should just go and shelter at my parents' house. Or find a local shelter. But that's just going to complicate matters. I need to talk to someone with legal knowledge. I have no idea where to even begin.

Last night, I prayed. I don't remember the last time I prayed in this way. I asked for a sign: "Help me find my way. Please..." Yana called for me. It was 5:30 a.m. I went to her room and laid next to her. She nudged her head close to me for comfort and fell back asleep as she had always done. She whispered in her dreamy state, 'Like in London,' and began to hum Winnie the Pooh'sTiddely Pom. That's the sign. London.

11 September, 2016

For the first time in my life, I am not going to censor this feeling. I will say it as it is. I will not be politically correct or try to be good...

I HATE HIM. I FUCKING DO.

How could he do this? How could he threaten me like that?

He said that if I did anything to secure work in London – even though he is the one forcing me to get a job to relief his financial pressure from a decision he made – he will divorce me and keep Yana. How dare he even say that to me, the fucking dickhead!

You know what else he said?

He said that if I was more curious about him, I would have realised he has changed. This asshole wanted me to take over being the provider but HIS WAY. He knows full well that in the best-case scenario, I would be making half of what he used to make in Corporate and would have to bear the additional costs of childcare and school fees that never existed in our expenses before. BUT that isn't even the point – the point was how he blamed me for his stress, how rude and arrogant he was, and how patronising and condescending.

I'm so blind.

He has always been like this. But I truly believed that what we had was worth sitting through the pain for. Even if it meant allowing myself to be treated in ways I would never have anyone else treat me... Unfortunately, I no longer believe this anymore.

Something has to change. I have tried everything in my capacity to shift things from within. It is not happening, it hasn't been happening, and in fact... it has gotten worse over time.

There is NO turning back.

I was directed by a lawyer who heard my predicament, to look into Relate and Women's Aid and the NSPCC websites. I completed the checklist, and I am shocked by the outcome because I never thought I was in an abusive relationship.

But the reality is this: he sees no reason for me to have my own money. He made sure I had no more savings. He threatened to keep Yana if I left him. He angrily blames me for his inability to have sex with me. He shuts me down in condescending and patronising ways when I say something 'wrong.' He withdraws information and affection to exclude and punish me. He puts me down and laughs it off. He corners my thinking with his interrogative or provocative approach that leads me to a dark doubtful place, defending my corner.

11 October, 2016

This is it. Brendon has received the divorce papers. He is seriously pissed off.

I am scared. He threatened to file a counter-claim. He threatened me to be prepared for litigation. He said he would not negotiate anything unless things resumed as they were before, i.e., Yana and I returned to the flat. He lied to the judge at the case conference, putting words in my mouth. He is being manipulative towards Yana.

In the same breath, he tells me I am the most important thing to him. He tells me we can work through our differences without getting divorced. I cannot trust him, and I do not want that mental torture anymore.

11 November, 2016

I am very disturbed. He had Yana on his lap watching the animation explainer video about premature ejaculation, repeatedly. I spoke to Diane who then went on to discuss within her circle of tutors, qualified therapists, and supervisors. Guess what she said:

What he's doing is not right and we would report it straight to child services. It's one thing to be neutral when you see children starting to explore, but it's another matter altogether to encourage. If you leave children to explore their sexuality (e.g., rubbing themselves against the bath ledge) that is one thing, but to send the message, 'you will please Daddy if you...' essentially is teaching the child to please Daddy in a certain sexual way. This can have serious repercussions on her psychological well-being later on. This is abuse; grooming of a 4-year-old who is not in a position to understand and make choices.

Google pods and sexual abuse. This is how perpetrators work. They put the blame on their victims in a bid to control them. This is a form of abuse. If you don't do something, you could be held as complicit in her abuse. It could well be the case that he is taking on the sexologist training place's beliefs wholesale, or it could be that he using them as justification for predatory behaviour to satisfy his own needs. If he is encouraging her to perform in front of him, that is very worrying. If you don't stop that, she will be far more fucked up and angry with you for not protecting her later than for calling the divorce. You need to get support behind you. I have spoken to two gestalt therapists and both are concerned about her safety, as am I.

The thing is, he is her dad. She is already fucked like that.

Diane used the word predatory – this is one of his kinks. What's confusing to me is that he seems like a great father. In fact, I believe he is very protective, and in this sense, I don't think he will consciously be abusive towards her. BUT, having said that, I found photos of her, that he took without my knowledge, some naked and some dressed in my clothes looking rather sexy... except she's a child. He also applauds her when she touches herself, and when she flashes her naked body or runs to him naked or pulls her bum cheeks apart to expose her asshole to him, laughing along for the laughter she generates. It has become a ritual somewhat, almost a secret Daddy and daughter agreement that it is starting to get me worried, especially when we split up and my presence will not be there to provide the counter-balance in the dynamic. I asked Brendon's tutor and this is what he wrote:

I have a very open and honest policy around children and sexuality – and even I was shocked that he was "encouraging and coaching her self-pleasure." That is NOT the parent's role. That implies the parent owns the child's sexual experiences and that is certainly NOT the case. Children have sexual rights – one is their privacy to explore without interference. You can eliminate shame and embarrassment and create a healthy sexual attitude from which a child can explore on their own terms by being neutral and matter of fact. Encouraging or even allowing her to touch his genitals is not healthy and doesn't demonstrate the importance of honouring personal boundaries and taking ownership of her own body. It's unlikely harm has been done yet, but if he continues this belief that it's his role to teach her to self-pleasure there could be. He needs a lot more education on this topic and to learn about personal boundaries.

We had a quick call after that. In a nutshell, there are educational materials for kids, and an adult explainer video about premature ejaculation, the giant vulva puppet pillows, pornographic and kink erotica materials, do not cut it for a toddler from a health and safety perspective.

I have to play this right. Safety is my priority. Brendon will never openly agree to do or not do anything, because to him, that would be complying to rules, which he hates, or tantamount to admitting wrong-doing; he will never see that as coming to an agreement or as a way of providing reassurance. I do not have enough hard evidence of abuse, sexual or otherwise. I have heard horror stories of victims losing custody because of insufficient evidence and blame-shifting. I definitely do not want to create any alarm or fear or shame or guilt, which would be totally unnecessary and could complicate matters for a young child even further. So, the sooner I can have Yana self-sufficient and aware about personal boundaries, the safer it will be for her, and the greater the chance for her to form a healthy boundary and relationship with Brendon, her father.

11 Months Trilogy (II)

11 January, 2017

Brendon's friend told me that my filing for divorce is an act of vindictiveness. He said that abuse is a matter of definition. In my moment of weakness, I felt awful. Then I realised, hang on a minute, I'm the one filing and wanting to leave. Who is he to tell me what my reasons for this are?

Letting go of self-doubt is perhaps one of the most difficult things for me to do in self-improvement.

Am I angry? Yes.

Am I vindictive? No.

Am I the one to blame for my own abuse? Hell, NO.

Why would I leave him to get back at him in revenge?

I may be weak, and because of who I am, Brendon can behave the way he did with me. BUT I did not cause Brendon to feel and act the way he has with me. So how can I be the cause of my being abused? That does not make sense. I sure as hell have gotten more clarity.

I have to give it to his friend though, that despite his judgments and beliefs, he caught himself and reverted to a coaching stance. He asked me two questions:

1. Is the sex good?
2. Do I like Brendon's energy?

My answer was No, on both counts. The answers came so clear and fast that I shocked myself. Inside, I felt so raw and so sad. Perhaps on seeing my glazed look, Brendon's friend offered a final statement:

Just be aware of feeling helpless.

Perhaps I had grown comfortable with feeling helpless. Perhaps I had been hiding behind that veil of innocence. It is time to grow into a whole a new level of being.

11 February, 2017

Brendon tried to make amends in his old ways. Through seduction and charm.

In the past, I would have gone running back. But I learnt over time, and especially in this instance, I feel as if there is nothing to return to. It felt final yet energetically I feel torn. Each time he is near, I feel pulled into the comfort of what I know and value; what I know to be the way we lived as a 'family,' and what I value, which is our 'family' unit. Each time he is near, I find it harder to be happy.

Whereas before I would receive his letters and song dedication with much hope and attachment-based love, all I feel now is the loss of hope, disappointment, and a detached form of love that flips so easily with anger.

He suggested a relationship coaching session with a therapist whom we both knew and trusted. I agreed and so a session was booked. But by the time the day arrived, I had already decided that I would move forward with the divorce. My hesitation was starting to show me the damage I would be bringing in. I feel clarity is so important, not just for myself, but for Yana. When I know from within me, I can be the stable one for her sense of security.

The lack of intimacy and affection that Brendon and I lived with on a daily basis, the animosity and finger-pointing that runs undercurrent when we were together, how we feel about and are affected by each other, would be what she picks up.

It is so hard to be subjected to his threats and have all these negative feelings about him, and witness Yana's innocent, loving interactions with him in utter duplicity. It is so difficult to be unaffected by his deep anger towards me that shows itself like a cold sociopath. How those charming eyes can look brutal and lethal towards me!

We faced the family court judge in a private case conference. It was surreal. My greatest fears all came true. Despite that, I am still in shock because I never thought he would say what he did about me... His words painted me as a criminal, and I'm not talking about just discrediting me as a mother. For the first time, I felt the pain of being accused of what I did and petrified by the cost of his words being believed more than mine. For the first time, I felt unfairness in a deep way... and how lost I was, blinded by my own shadows that I had confused to be my light.

There's a part of me that rings, "what have I done?" while another part of me rings, "it's not my fault." There's a voice that screams, "I was pushed here," while another voice screams back, "I take charge." There's much noise in silence and there is much silence in noise. I need to get out of my head and out of the painful state.

11 March, 2017

I wanted to get out of my head and my painful state, and I received so many prompts to dance. It's amazing what comes when I open myself up to receiving help. I sat down to do a meditation and it turns out that at the end of that session, there was a dance. I lay down to sleep and I tuned into music that awoke the dancer within me up. I listened to music and I heard words to do with dance.

So, my dear guardian angels, I hear you! I will dance.

OMG, you won't believe this. I just received news that Jem (sacred dance teacher) is in town and I have just been asked if I want to co-facilitate one of the journeys she will be leading! I am so excited! Since this storm with Brendon began, I have felt like my life is somewhat 'hanging.' I have not danced properly for a while and I really miss it. I have not had much inspiration to, but it looks like the time is now!

I'm sure dancing again will help me with the divorce counselling and mediation process. Every time I walk in there, I feel like I am the defendant instead of the plaintiff. After every session, no doubt I feel less doubtful about the divorce, but I doubted who I am and what I stand for that bit more than before the session, and definitely feel more anxious about the flipside happening to my vision of a bright future.

Brendon wanted me to rewrite all my grounds for

divorce to a language that fits him. There's a part of me that feels it is already so vague and watered down yet he has the cheek to make me state that my grounds for divorce is because of my perception.

As Brigit says, "Abuse is abuse."

Even if there are varying degrees of it.

But I did not want to stay in that state of blame, and neither did I want to risk losing custody if he puts up an argument in defence that I am mentally unstable. Who cares if he also says he is proud of me and that I'm doing an amazing job as a mum albeit at the cost of our marriage? Who cares if he apologises for withdrawing sex and intimacy from me to punish me? His logical, deductive ways are far more believable than a verbal account of abuse in forms not yet recognised by the law. There are so many horror stories of abuse claims being overturned due to lack of evidence and blame-shifting, with the resulting outcome devastating to all concerned, not just the abused. I cannot bring myself to make the claims because I am afraid of what will happen if I did.

Brigit's words are in my mind: "Just because you have a high tolerance of poor behaviour that is non-physically evident does not mean that he did not do what he did."

If I were stronger to begin with, I might never have 'built' this blue monster of a bully, I might never have attracted him nor have been attracted to him in the first place...

Speaking of blue monsters, Mum brought me this huge cookie, which is sitting in front of me now, reminding me of the Cookie Monster in Sesame Street. I might just have had my innocent childhood wish to see the Cookie Monster every day inadvertently come true!

CTRL-ALT-DELETE please.

Reboot. I don't want Cookie Monster anymore. Please take it back.

Wait. Did I just reinforce that by not wanting it?

Haha, I'd better go and dance!

11 April, 2017

Co-facilitating the sacred dance with Jem was a God-send.

There was a point in the journey where I unexpectedly felt the presence of Archangel Michael; unexpected because the spirit guide who I called to be with me was Ixchel and her energy was there throughout. Not only was this a bonus from an experiential perspective, the visual was remarkably helpful and truthful.

I never knew about the visions of Archangel Michael until I looked it up after my astounding experience. Archangel Michael has reportedly showed up like a vacuum cleaner sucking out dark or heavy energy in order for people to shine their inner light even brighter.

In my vision, Archangel Michael came down to me from like a knight charging towards me full of light, swiftly yet in a reassuring way with a sword. However, when he was above my head, he put his hand of light, not the sword, into me from the crown of my head right to the base of my spine, swiped, and stayed there to draw and channel all scattered dark spots in me upwards back into the skies from my crown. I have never seen anything like this, let alone experienced the 'cleansing' effect of such an intervention!

By the end of it, I felt light, but I walked with some level of disbelief... there was something so real and surreal, so new. I arrived home feeling foggy-headed, and got a call from Brendon, which I did not welcome, and did not know how to respond to. In my effort to clear some head space, I popped to the corner shop and found a deck of Archangel Michael Oracle cards, so I bought them.

I asked just one question – what do I need to know, right now?

The card I picked was:

"It's time to leave this unhealthy situation."

I say no more.

11 May, 2017

I got off a call with Inez a couple of hours ago. One thing about going through a divorce is that I have discovered the amount of support I have around me. I feel very blessed. I receive a lot of suggestions aimed at helping me. I never ask for much, but I guess on some level, I must be asking it, which is why people say what they say to me.

It seems as if I had unconsciously been asking for more fun. Perhaps I was sick and tired of going into my thinking head, rehashing legal proceedings that overlay the future canvas. Every minute was spent in as productive, fulfilling and good feeling ways as possible... but it is not how I would feel when I have fun. Having fun feels more carefree and flowing with laughter that works my jaw and belly muscles tired from the natural breathwork it triggers.

Anyway, Inez and I were talking about dating websites. The reason being, she found that dating helped her through the entire process of her divorce – to have fun, to get the male contact, to feel her sex appeal and physically move into her future space instead of standing on the divorce iceberg floating to the promised land.

I'm not convinced. Last month, I went for a dinner organised by a millennial start-up co-founder and met a consultant who worked in technology. I got into a very engaging conversation with him about work, when all of a sudden, he threw me a curve ball and asked, 'Are you dating?'

It turns out, the event was marketed to another group this same founder was also co-founder of, which was an online dating group. I was lost for words for that split second, and as if my world went in slow motion, I suddenly noticed that he was actually quite good looking, and I was flattered that he was interested in me in that way.

We went for a date, and I loved every bit of the 'gentleman and lady' orchestration, where he arranged everything, from the first meeting point through to the dinner venue, giving me enough time to get back for my train, and allowing me to relax into being looked after like a princess. I felt like a movie star!

But, there was an awkwardness in that I felt like I was being interviewed and it killed the chemistry that could have been there. There was hardly any flirtation for a date and the attraction index kind of went flat. Despite that, I liked that we were on the same page from a date perspective.

I checked out the website he was on, and when I saw the form they each had to fill out and photos they had to upload, I got doubtful. The profiling assumed that I know what I'm about, I know what I want, and I disclose fully all that I know about myself and what I'm looking for in a life partner.

Mind you, this is much sleeker than some others I had seen when Brendon went on them. It seems like the selective pool of membership, the extensive profiling, and the transparency and high touch approach, meant that folks only out for finding a sex partner are filtered out.

When Brendon was on dating websites, I read what he wrote, and I read what some of our mutual acquaintances whom we spotted on the platform wrote... and it feels different from who they are in person. From these experiences, I'm not convinced. But my dear friends kept telling me about social experiments and circular dating and not to take it so seriously. Yet I still cannot see myself going on a dating website!

11 June, 2017

I cannot believe it – I finally managed to have lunch with Brendon one-to-one. There was nothing left to talk about, nothing left to argue about, and with reduced anxiety over fears of saying the wrong thing that could cause problems in court, we could simply be. Having said that, I remember letting my guard down and reverted to sharing my feelings, and immediately, Brendon hooked on it, and began his 'deductive,' 'directive,' 'therapeutic' style of conversing with me. Having been apart for a while now, I immediately spotted it. The difference is that this time when it happened, I looked at him in the eye and without any angst or frustration, smiled and said, 'you just did it again.' Brendon's face clocked the difference in my response.

I had mentioned this to him before on several occasions… how he would turn every 'problem' or 'emotion' I share with him, back to me... which is helpful, if not for the fact that he had vested interest for me to respond in a particular way that suited him.

He did say to me once, 'I know what you mean, Kerry. I can understand why you want a divorce. I just don't think that divorce is the way to solve our problem. You're destroying our family and Yana's life.'

I beg to differ. I see another path, a more hopeful and fulfilling one but it involves taking a step into the big unknown and it's challenging traditions and long-standing beliefs. I firmly replied, 'If you believe so, if you hold an intention to prove you're right, if you pay attention to all the things that are wrong according to your beliefs, she'll be left with no choice but to live up to your expectations.'

I looked him straight in the eyes and started to get all teary-eyed. My heart, however, was wailing, desperate for comfort. Eventually, I will learn how to give this comfort to my heart all on my own.

Since then, there were several more occasions where I had forgotten how it was like to be psycho-ed in an intense heady debate and opened up the opportunity for Brendon to do just that. But it's all good because I am reminded with greater fervour, each time, why I chose this path and why I would not have done it another way.

You know what I feel like doing?

Letting my hair down and running with the sexiest running gear possible along the beach, all on my own, protected by the watching stars, and screaming, laughing, and dancing in celebration at the end of it, complete with flowers, fire, and fragranced water.

The weeks of mediation are coming to a formal close. In a couple of weeks, the interim judgment will be passed, and I am hugely relieved! And happy! My heart is open and my floodgates too. One big mountain has been surpassed and I am about to step onto new land.

I never knew the smell of freedom could taste so magical until this day!

11 July, 2017

I am officially divorced… and to celebrate this, I have arrived in a new town with large suitcases and a child in tow. The smell and taste of freedom drowned my exhaustion as I looked forward to a new beginning. I felt my whole being was lighter. I felt freer. I felt hopeful. I felt excited. I wanted to dance!

There is no better reason to celebrate. Oh, how funny, just as I wrote celebrate, I noticed a poster right above me:

Pizza Express Soho Open Mic

10 August 2017 @ 8pm

I'm going! For definite! It's a sign!

That gives me time to sort out childcare, and fingers crossed, find us a proper flat. The airbnb is alright, but it's a big house share and a mouse showed up in the kitchen last night. The guy who runs this place, Fred, is a budding musician, I wonder if he would be interested in this Open Mic?

11 August, 2017

I have been smiling and feeling super alive for most of today, which is almost embarrassing. I still cannot believe what happened. So Fred decided to do the Open Mic. We went together. I have never heard or seen him perform like this before. Whenever he practiced at home, it all sounded muffled and I never saw his expression. He is super-duper HOT. And his body, OMFG! It seriously reminded me of Ryan Gosling's character in Stupid Crazy Love, in one of his scenes with Emma Stone, where she went, "Seriously, it's like you're Photoshop-ed!"

I don't think I have ever been "taken" the way I had been taken last night. It was CRAZY shit. I mean, we weren't even drinking much. The high was natural, triggered by his performance, and the joy afterwards, walking home together under the starry sky on a mild, almost warm evening. It was a big surprise because there was hardly any physical contact before, during and after his performance. But we just talked and laughed, and when we got home, we went straight to Fred's room to listen to the latest demo he had just cut the day before. It was that elegant and pumping music that a couple of sips of champagne simply accentuated. And he just came for me. I couldn't help myself. I had my period, so it was all rather messy and I did tell him but he wasn't bothered at all.

I felt quite self-conscious, as it has been forever since I had sex, let alone being so sexually desired and attracted, and the combination was lethal. Even as I write now, I can feel my face flush and I'm getting wet... embarrassingly so. What fascinates me is how our insecurities showed up that night. There I was all worried that my vagina was too loose, without a clue that he was feeling intimidated in the same moment. When I asked if he had slept with a woman who has had a child before, and he said no, I asked how he felt about it, and his answer was, 'a little shy because you have more experience.' I was dumbfounded.

I didn't see him at all in the morning, and when I asked to play the piano, he said he had a lot of work. Then he came back, showered, and left the house. I have a strange feeling he is avoiding me, especially as I leave tomorrow...

11 September, 2017

So, Fred has gone silent. It has been one month now. Nada. I just learnt a new word – ghosting.

I can't believe it. No man has ever done this to me before. Or perhaps I have been protected mostly. I'm finding this hard to deal with. It baffles and confuses me.

Diane shared a wonderful post on Facebook about this, and how serendipitous that I read it today! Hormones bond the woman to the man she slept with for a good while, and for many woman, the act of penetrative sex involves the receiving of a man inside, which forces up trust. To have that not acknowledged makes ghosting so yucky.

I have to say I'm proud of myself for walking into a bar all on my own, with baby Yana fast asleep and safe at Kiki's. I realise that I would never have done something like this before. I had a proper conversation with the barman, got another drink on the house, and didn't feel sad or desperate. I did have to resist looking at my phone because I found it hard to just sit, sip, and stare into space!

There was this Irish guy who had a bit too much to drink, who started chatting me up, but I have to give it to him because he said it'd be good to meet up for coffee and have a proper conversation when he's sober.

Nonetheless, I caught myself thinking about Fred every now and then. Sometimes in disappointment, other times in laughter, because imagine for a moment that whatever that you conjure up in your mind is created, only in a different dimensional reality… If that were the case then technically, this movie that I'm producing is happening there and then.

I forgot how emotionally connected I feel with a man I slept with, until Fred came onto the scene. I never thought it would turn out this way either. I am flattered that he has seen all of me right from the beginning, because we shared the house, he has seen me at my best and worst, with and without make up, dressed up and dressed down, and he has seen me as a mum, as a friend, as a host, as a girl... And he found me, in his words, very attractive and sexy.

With Fred, the intimacy deepened that night in the room, and perhaps that was what scared him off! He shared so much about himself, his past, his stories, his struggle, his insecurities, his challenges, and his hopes.

11 October, 2017

That Irish guy turned out to be a bit of a dickhead. We were supposed to meet at an event. He did not show up on time. By the time he arrived, Kiki and I had left for a club where we met a rather secretive but straightforward American born Chinese businessman. Irish guy showed up there, having tracked me down. Not only did he gate crash, he drank my drink, and his octopus hands started exploring!

Business man and Kiki intervened, and when he would not leave, security was called and Irish guy was escorted out for harassment. The next day, he was massively apologetic and wanted to make up for it. I was curious and said I could meet him after the farewell drinks. He made up for it with an expensive dinner at one of the poshest restaurants in Mayfair, and he got us a private area in perhaps the coolest cocktail bar there after dinner. The next day, he asked if I wanted to go to his house for 'cuddles.'

It turns out this guy is 15 years younger than me! I don't blame him for trying, but I was not born yesterday, and I certainly am not getting involved in bed with someone I do not know.

But that night out with Kiki was something to remember – we had a whale of a time! I don't remember when I last had such a girly crazy dancing night. After the Irish guy incident, the ABC businessman escorted us to a membership club, where we danced until the lights came on. I had zero chemistry with him even though we danced and talked and got along... and I must have been living on another planet because when lights came on, he asked if I wanted to go back to his room with him. I responded calmly, 'No'. And he left. I did not feel any sexual tension at all with him, and in fact, at one point, I even thought he was gay!

Kiki and I ended up in McDonalds where we met Joe and Alex, who joined us at our table, self-invited. They were both very handsome. I met Joe a week later and sussed out he was also 15 years younger than me, but I still gave him some airtime because we had some interesting conversations. That Irish guy was a wealthy trader in comparison to Joe who is a security guard on hourly rates. The former did not buy me a drink, came to my table and drank my drink, then practically molested me until security was called. Joe bought us a bottle to share with what looked like his last 20 quid, walked me home, and called me afterwards. He wanted to know everything about me and he even wanted to meet Yana. But that was what sent my alarm bells ringing. I knew then that I did not want to be in a relationship with Joe. These are boys. The phase of life they are at is not what I need for the long haul. I think if he did not move towards wanting a relationship, we could have grown platonically, but given where we are at in life, it was better to be clear about where I stood and draw the line.

I joked that there must be a vibe that I'm sending out, flattering as it is to believe that I look at least 15 years younger. And I thought Fred who was nine years younger was young (bad) enough. But I honestly noticed that it has to do with something triggering in my mind since I read those Deepak Chopra books... *Ageless Body Timeless Mind,* and *Super Genes...* I've concluded that the concept of age is created out of the innate human need to create, and aging is largely conditioned.

It seems as if the minute attention was moved away from age, it was no longer a barrier for me to do something new, get divorced or have a child, a fountain of youth sprang from a fresh bed of grass. I have realised that, the clearer I was about what I wanted, the more playful I could be and the more attractive I became. BUT, I don't think that my vibe-ing what I want has manifested in physical form in the way I envisage!

Someone once said to me that following one's desire leads to adventure. I have no doubt this is true. There is so much room to grow in terms of riding this adventure though. There is a balance that can be struck between staying and moving; staying makes you brave, moving makes you strong. The more I call out what's not said, the more I call out the energy, the greater the clarity between parties, such that the space expands to facilitate new movement.

11 November, 2017

Out of the blue, three months since he ghosted me, Fred texted me to go out the next time I was in town. I flipped. In a nice way.

Hey, thanks for asking. I've been in town a lot but figured you were busy. By the way, I don't sleep with any guy, and when I do, I want a bit of respect. Disappearing the way you did was not cool.

His reply was, 'okay.' That was it… one word.

Some minutes later, he text: 'You didn't like sex with me?'

Can you believe it?

So, I played along: 'Are you crazy? With that super-hot body, why not?'

Fred replied: 'Because I come too fast. It's a problem. For some it's ok, some not.'

In the past, with the ex, who had premature ejaculation as well, he would blame me. He would have said I did it wrong, I spoiled the fun, I made him come too quick, I made it too mechanical and physical only, etc. And being young and naive, I believed every word. Until I grew up.

But it's odd that the first guy I slept with after my ex was one who suffers from Premature Ejaculation too. Perhaps it's more common than I thought.

Last week, I met Robin, who works as a Shaman at a gathering he hosted in the yoga community here. I loved the dance and breathwork, and it reminded me of what I missed in my spiritual circle... my spiritual brothers and sisters... the warm, fuzzy feeling and comfort of long hugs and long eye gazes.

We hung out a couple of days ago, and I asked: "How do you deal with erotic transference?"

"What do you mean?"

"You work with a lot of women, at an intimate level... I'm sure there are many women who would 'fall in love' with you, and you may want to sleep with some of them in the process."

Robin took a deep breath and blew it out with a loud sheesh, put his hands around my waist as if we were slow dancing without music, and as we moved with the energy, he looked me deep in the eye and said, "I've learnt to really honour the women. Instead of just 'consuming,' the way the energy might feel like as it takes form in the physical body... to hold space, and really see and honour the woman."

We didn't have sex. It would have been too easy to go down that path, yet it was not too difficult to hold back. There was something sacred in that moment… the connection felt Divine, the sexual impulse transformed in vibe. There was an ability to look after what was present, what was shared, what was hoped for or fantasised about, and to let it all go.

11 Months Trilogy (III)

11 January, 2018

My highlight for January must be my encounter with Tony.

I met Tony at Jason's leaving party, and we had the most serendipitous of conversations as we gravitated more and more towards each other throughout the evening. It was crazy, the timing of our life crisis, the things we cared about, excitement about our dreams. The contact dance was remarkably seductive, passionate and free flowing. And the run out to get supper and into the freezing cold winter night to find a place to cuddle was oh-so-romantic. Our banters were totally funny as we cracked each other up laughing. As fate would have it, we could not have sex that night, despite all the lustful, alcohol exaggerated sexual impulse to do so. We simply messed around as I went into my head telling myself not to mess this up because I really fancied him; as they say, don't sleep with a guy you fancy on the first date, no matter how hot.

He tried to guess my age. After Fred, Joe and the Irish dude, I wasn't surprised to learn that Tony is ten years younger than me, and I have to admit that I was rather disappointed, even though compared to fifteen years younger, this was an improvement! I'm guessing that my lively little girl spirit, the one who does not care about age, is drawing guys who find that lively little girl spirit attractive.

What I did not expect, after such a deeply meaningful and fun evening together, was total silence as to what it all meant, especially not after how we took a moment to look into the mirror at our naked bodies as if it was a photograph, and how we said goodbye.

I had a chat with Jason about it after he cheekily asked how things went with Tony, encouraging me to call. It must be a generational thing, but I don't see calling a guy the morning after as an attractive thing to do. I made a point though, that I was disappointed in Tony, and I think it's partly because I expected more from a man, and partly because I had never been "ghosted" before until Fred. I am realising, the game has changed, and I'm no longer the same person in the singles field. I'm a divorced single mom who is turning 41.

Jason, being the loving friend that he is, intervened. Without his intervention, I don't think this January encounter would have happened. Tony texted.

Hey Kerry,

Jason mentioned to me just now that he got the impression you were expecting me to call. So in this message, I want to lovingly share with you where I stand. It was really great to meet and dance together and I'd love to meet up in the new year and continue the multiple conversations we started ;-). However, I also want to be honest about where I stand, especially since you have a daughter. I do not want to create any expectations that this will lead to a serious relationship. However, I am super curious to spend more time together and see where our bodies take us. Please feel free to share your thoughts. I was going to share this in person when we met but Jason suggested for me to write first. Hope this is okay and we can meet as planned in Jan. Tx

I replied:

Hi, morning!

Sorry for the delay in reply. Was holding a global meditation space and the full moon was so intense I crashed out by the end. Thank you for the beautiful message. I love Jason so much. The conversation came up with him as he asked me to call you, etc, and move things forward, as he was surprised you didn't call. Perhaps he sees something we don't. I didn't expect a call to be honest, but a text to acknowledge what was shared and call the energy out. In any case, I liked you and what we shared was special. I just felt it odd to not touch on it and move as if nothing happened. Let me sit with this rainbow elephant for now.

Tony texted back to say, "Rainbow elephant is a lovely way to put it!"

A few days later, I told him that the rainbow elephant had spoken. I said that I wished to share honestly and whatever comes as a result, I am not attached to and have no fear, and I invited him to do the same:

First, I am open about the form my path takes in life. Relationships fascinated me but my foreground today is energetic manifestation through purity of intent. This is my journey and my work now.

Which leads me to share that I have a deep respect for the primal forces of creation. My human side is dancing with great honour as it learns respect for the sexual energy between Masculine and Feminine, both intra and interpersonal lyrics. This work that begun in 2015, is still spiralling through in beauty.

Therefore, I appreciate where you stand and have no issues with that. I hold you in equal esteem, and what I experienced as avoidance as a way of coping (whether from men in general, from you specifically, or how I responded), I am now asked to shift, to call out and face, grow in independence and strength, and mirror de-conditioning, restructuring, and co-creation.

The connections we share represent for me bold courage in living new paradigms moving through to open this space, and for that alone, I am grateful. I am super curious about where the creative energy will lead to what is being co-created in profoundly magical ways.

It is no coincidence that all these weaving of stories and parallels, and soulful insights are arising at this time, almost simultaneously, for many of us hooked up to the web of light while remaining connected to Mother Earth. We are here for each other in capacities that align with love, with who we are. And with this, comes stepping up and growing in multidimensional ways. It means holding space in ways that include the sacredness of human experience to allow for flow... to allow wellness to come from energies of love.

On that note, I look forward to our dialogue in January. I trust things will unfold as Divinely orchestrated and humanly facilitated as probable. Keep me posted about dates and timings. We can spend a couple of nights together.

Some weeks after, Tony arrived, and we had the funniest

most engaging conversations over dinner, talking and laughing, before adjourning to a local pub nearby to carry on talking late into the night. Walking back hand-in-hand in the cold winter night transported me back to the fun night out, as if we went back to a timestamp in a movie, to continue where we left off. This time, we took the contact dance to the bedroom and it wasn't long before we got rolling and taking off clothes... and that was when it started to get a bit much for me.

I felt like I was being devoured, taken by a wild animal. There was something really primal about it, and at first, it all felt very natural and pleasurable... BUT, soon, it also got painful... Fear kicked in, and when my words, "Stop it, you're hurting me" fell on deaf ears, I got nervous. The good news was that, all of a sudden, Yana called for me and I went to attend to my dear baby and dozed off. When I woke up, I noticed two mugs with coffee granules, a kettle full of fresh boiled water, and a sleeping Tony on the sofa; he had fallen asleep waiting for me.

I went to shower, and to my horror, I saw patchy swollen bruises all over my body, my arms in particular. And as the water hit my raw skin, I felt tears streaming down my cheeks even though I had no tears from the numbing shock of realising what had just taken place.

The next day, we still spent all day together, talking, but I noticed I was more distant and reflective in my own bubble, and he was his usual chatty self, but having accomplished his mission, there was no longer any flirtation, no more playfulness from attraction driven by sexual tension. But hormones got me, I think, because I still wanted to be physically close to him... Not because

I wanted more sex, but I enjoyed the intimacy of touch, and I think we both wanted and welcomed that – cuddling and snuggling with a movie and a brief chat before saying goodnight and goodbye.

In the days that followed, he was on my mind a lot, but as he disappeared the way he did before, and as I looked at my body each and every day when I showered, I knew this marked the end of our intimacy. Getting to know him has been intense, quite like a bootcamp, and it felt intimate because he shared a lot, not just in words, but also in how he carried himself, his swift walk, his nods, his curious mind, his deep searching eyes... and I felt my heart opening up a nurturing space for him. I felt him giving permission to himself for showing me his wild side, and for giving me permission to hit him in the face if it all got too messy for me! The friendship, this micro-relationship as he calls it, never developed further though, which saddened me somewhat, perhaps just as a part of parting ways.

Did sex spoil the friendship? I don't think so. The nature of this friendship, the tone of it, the connected-disconnection, the fear and desire interplay, assured that it could only be fleeting. Not many would enjoy dragging or being dragged along nor to make space to reflect, learn and debrief with the person they just slept with, and it appears that this was the dynamic that stood out. Perhaps this is the bit that keeps the vulnerability out of the picture, and to take the experience for what it is.

I don't know how people can get into intimate circular dating. I don't think the way my body responds from a hormone perspective would change, so I probably would have had to desensitize myself from feeling empty once the man goes off disconnected. I'm not sure if desensitizing is what I want either. I told Kiki about this and she got really angry. She is super protective. She made me promise not to see him ever again, and though somewhat sceptical, she was pleased that I had blocked his number on my phone and social media accounts.

11 February, 2018

I met Dev, who works in publishing, at a tapas night in mid-December. The coincidence led to some interesting conversation. He was friendly and Brigit and I had fun laughing throughout the 20-minute exchange. BUT, by the end of it, he was "pushing it" and totally stole kisses that it pissed us off. Nevertheless, he invited us to ski and messaged soon after as well, saying that he would be in contact when he returns from travel, which he did. He asked me to meet him for drinks after work, to which I said okay for 7-ish, and guess what his reply was?

"Trouble is, I only live here during the week for work and head off to Brighton at the weekends! I'm more than happy to take you out for a drink tonight if it's okay to crash on your sofa for the night?"

You have GOT to be JOKING!

I do not know this person at all. Why would anyone in their sober and sane mind agree to a total stranger sleeping overnight after drinks?

I replied simply, "I see. I'm sorry. Another time then :)"

"I could meet you for 1 or 2 drinks at 7pm then head off to Brighton if that's good with you? Be great to see you again x"

At this point, I have to admit, this quick turnaround he

attempted, backfired. The following week, he text again, "How was your weekend? Are you free to meet tonight? X"

"Hey, this is not a good week, sorry. You ought to look up my friend for company. She's single and childless so less planning and more social calendar than mine perhaps."

"I messaged her on Facebook. What's her number? Can you tell her to call me? X"

"Nay, boundaries. She will reply if and when she is ready."

"Boundaries, ha! Are you secret agents?"

"Let's just say that I'm too much trouble for you :)"

"Why? I like a challenge x ha"

"I sense you prefer to chill, no planning ahead headache, no deep conversations etc..."

Next day, he text: "Can you talk? What time are you back? Fancy a drink after work?"

Does this guy hear me when I say that I cannot do last minute?

"Have plans already. Sorry."

"Okay, don't forget to pass my number to your friend!"

Next day, he text again, "Fancy a drink?"

"You might be let down as I just decided to give up alcohol for Lent. Happy to have something non-alcoholic and warm."

"I'm warm and non-alcoholic X ha"

Next day, he text again, "Drinks tonight?"

Can you believe that?

Which part of "I don't do last minute as I have childcare

to plan for" does he not get?

A week later, he sent a couple of texts again!

"How are you? Are you free to meet for a drink tonight? X"

And he left me a voice message.

I replied the next day:

"Hey, sorry if texts got confusing. First, last week, I did say I couldn't make it and you still texted on the day itself. Secondly, sorry if this is broken record, I can hardly ever make on-the-day arrangements due to child care. We're in totally different phases of life. Hope you got company in the end. Best wishes."

"Call me and we can talk darling XX and arrange to meet. "

A week later, he text, "Are you free to meet tonight? X"

OH, MY FUCKING GOD!

A week later, he text, "I have a spare VIP ticket for the Rag n Bone gig at Alexander Palace tonight, if you want to come with me? Dev X"

A week later, he text this, "How are you? X"

I continued to ignore him. It was time to end the moronic text exchanges.

This incident reminded me of Rob or Will... This guy (yes, he is just one guy) asked for my phone number at the toilet doors, while he was on a first date with someone he had just met on Tinder, with a different name from what he signed off as in his text. When I asked, he said I could call him Will, or Sir.

Dodgy. He was also totally off-grid, so there was no way of sussing out his background. Two days after the intro texts, this was the exchange, believe it or not:

Rob or Will:

"What you been up to?"

Me:

"Just done putting my daughter to bed."

"Ah ok... I was having my birthday meal. Shall I pop over? haha."

YOU ARE KIDDING ME?! These guys must live on a different planet...

Me:

"Happy birthday! Unless you're from BT, my abode is closed to strangers. Sorry."

Rob or Will:

"That's ok."

Two days later:

"Are you free for a drink sometime?"

Me:

"Yes"

The next day:

"When are you free?"

"Depends on where, London or local?"

"Local. Now? I'm at the Crown already."

"Can't do now I'm afraid."

A few hours later...

"Come see me x"

"In PJs about to sleep. Need more notice. Have a little one to care for. It's been a long day."

":(wanna see you x"

Me, copy and pasted:

"In PJs about to sleep. Need more notice. Have a little one to care for. It's been a long day. Night."

":(night"

Then a month later:

"I was in Crown with you haha... but you were with your daughter so I didn't want to say hi :)"

"Why not? I did see someone who looked like you with two kids."

Rob or Will:

"Haha definitely not me! Was with my brother."

Then a month later, when I was having drinks with a gay friend:

"I'm sitting opposite you."

"Come say hello, sorry I can't remember very well how you look."

"LOL, forget it."

The next day, he text:

"Would have been awkward. Was that your boyfriend?"

By this time, I couldn't resist poking him because I told him very early on, I don't do texts when it comes to getting to know a person:

"Don't think so, not awkward for me. He's someone who took my number and asked me out to get to know me, cos I don't do texts, remember? ;)"

"You like two men at the same time? Haha, how did it go?"

"I like people, yes, and I love meaningful conversations."

"Answer my question. That's how a conversation works, right? ;) "

"No, that's how interrogation works :)"

And that was the end of the text messaging with this Shady Sir.

11 March, 2018

This morning at 3 a.m., I was woken up by a chant playing in my mind: Chidananda Rupa Shivoham Shivoham. I remember the first time the image of Christ came to me, about ten years ago. I was lying in Victoria Park on a sunny day. I must have dozed off, but the next thing I knew, an extraordinary bright light shone down on me and as I tried to get a good look at what it was. It was Jesus Christ. Imagine my shock! I was raised without religion in a religious country, I never resonated with Christianity, and I was disillusioned by religious door-to-door sales people who called themselves missionaries and told me that if I believed in Christ I would get to Heaven.

Last year was the first time in my entire life that I celebrated Christmas day in church. My tears flowed throughout the service. I was filled with joy as part of me heard and understood something that all the human noise had drowned out.

I kept up with my 40-day self-upgrade protocol, which included fasting, still and movement meditation, and daily walks in nature. Halfway through, I had a dream that this bright light swirled and took the form of a masculine entering me as my spine curved upwards, pushing my belly button towards the sky and back down. The stream of energy flowing through me seemed to draw my limbs and body as if they were antennas picking up information of various frequencies, as if I was receiving the answers to all my questions. The pulse quickened as my entire body vibrated. I felt like I was being pulled into another world. I remember wondering if I was dying. Then my entire sacral began to dance and my breath quickened to gasping rate as I felt it peak into what seemed like orgasmic pleasure. It was so real and I only realised it was a dream when my eyes opened to the blinking light of a YouTube subscription notification on my phone.

Atlantean transmission.

I thought, what is that?

So, I put on my headset, and as the images became more and more vivid, tears of homecoming streamed and streamed. There was so much light, love, and beauty.

I woke up finding joy in everything, laughing at the simplest of life's activities, and seeing everything dance with me.

I woke up with such clarity about my true heart's desires, with a deep knowing that for me, it is far more interesting, potent, and expansive to focus and devote my intimate relationship with one person in a human experience. There was no logic nor debate about attraction, polyamory, kink... and that for me, conscious monogamy with an open mind and a loving heart flows well and rings true with my being, at least at this point in time.

I felt the presence of my life partner in an instant, even though my human mind cannot comprehend this, because in my human relationships, this spot is an open position. Overnight, I felt such curiosity, fun, and wonder. Who could this be?

It was even more fun as I realised I have zero sense of

urgency because I finally learnt how to be in my Feminine and receive the holding love of the Masculine, from the world I design, without needing to see it, touch it, and feel it, in a physical way. Yet, I am super-duper excited about this impending meeting, for I know it is there. I can feel it, taste it, and smell it. I cannot wait for him to arrive and for us to recognise each other. And I wonder how we will each know.

11 April, 2018

I'm laughing inside as I write this. I can't believe that a simple encounter can feel so joyful, free and flowing. This morning, there I was, standing on the train platform and as I turned to look at the arrival times, 11:11 flashed on the display. I was about to meet a stranger I connected online with in February through an international community of people who appreciate the fine life. We arranged to meet as we would both be in Jakarta at the same time.

I remember thinking, 'new beginning,' walking through a portal into the foundation of family, and concluding in wonder – is this guy going to be the one?

As fate would have it, he was not. LOL!

BUT, I reckon that I indeed walked through a portal more ceremoniously than before. I also feel strongly that because I had so much fun and laughter, this is precisely what my answer is for now. I need fun and laughter, even more than I need a man.

In the past, I would have judged my time with meeting Marc as frivolous and a total waste of time. I would have judged him as perverted and I would have played the innocent one. I would have judged my playfulness at lunch time today as slutty and I would not have been able to relate with Marc in equal measure and a good dose of light-heartedness!

He asked, "When was the last time you dated?"

I said, "What do you mean by dating? To me, dating is like meeting new people, making new friends, and learning about them. In this case, because I am a woman who likes men, then it is learning about new male friends I meet, in view of spending more of my time with them to potentially build a life together. So, with this definition, then I'm dating all the time!"

Marc laughed a determined laugh.

"I mean, it seems like it's been a while... how do you get your needs met? I mean, how long has it been since you had sex?"

I thought to myself, "A-ha, this is what he means by dating!"

"Take a guess."

"Six months," Marc muttered with penetrating eyes.

I smiled with pride, stared back into his eyes, and without an ounce of fear, said, "Ah... nope!"

"Damn, it was less than that, wasn't it?"

"You're trying to get me into bed, aren't you?"

"Yes," Marc replied, laughing.

"I don't really do one-night stands. Been there, done that. Not my thing anymore."

"Well, it would be a one-day stand! Come join me for a massage then dinner and sky bar."

"That's inviting, but I can't as I have to get home for my daughter. But, thank you!"

"Just come to the sky bar tonight then."

"I'm out with my friend, but if she can be convinced to drive downtown, then maybe."

I had a wonderful lunchtime, very chilled, bantering and laughing away. He seemed charming, funny, smart, well-travelled, honest, and open-minded. I loved our exchange about culture, and we laughed about cultural differences in greeting people with a kiss or two or three or four! And he definitely knows how to work his money to draw attraction in such an elegant way.

We exchanged a few texts.

"Just to say, I appreciate your laughter and the lunch earlier. Thank you so much!"

"I was thinking of texting you the same thing... I loved meeting you and the time we spent together! I'm meeting my friend for dinner at 20:00 but later he won't join me as he has an early flight. I hope you can come to the sky bar xxx"

"I won't make it to the sky bar tonight, I'm afraid. My friend is sleeping off a flu, and I'm travelling at 8 a.m. tomorrow. If you do feel like coming to this side of the neighbourhood, then I'm happy to go with you to a cocktail bar here, if you pick me up on your way. By the way, are you sure you're not from Montenegro?"

"Actually, I have to work for about 30 min more and when I finish... 30/40 mins of car is a bit too much! I would love to meet you but it seems that you don't... Oh, and it is said that Italians kiss twice and I always give two kisses."

I thought to myself, "A-ha, guilt tripping!"

"I getcha, self-care is important! And I think I did alright in Maths? xxx is 3 crosses right?"

"Yes, but in reality, I always give 2! ;)"

"Hmmmmm, what is Reality...? I could never have a

relationship with you! ;)"

"Who knows! Leave free your energy... ;)"

"Oh, for sure, energy always flowing, and deeply respect it. It's the force of life. Powerful. And I take my power responsibly, haha ;)"

"LOL :-D So… do I have a chance to see you at the Sky Bar? I understood that you were not able to meet me because you had to meet your friend but at this point..."

"I was supposed to be out... but it's me on my own now, sleepy from childcare and still home in gym clothes. Not the best idea to rush down in a Grabcar on my own this late. Plus, two sexy people getting together this late spells trouble for tomorrow!"

"I actually love a beautiful girl in gym clothes. Remember... life needs to be lived/enjoyed, and trouble sometimes can be very fun/good memories! ;)

PS: Thanks for the sexy... "

"Haha, I getcha, totally, maybe that's why part of me is choosing an alternative reality ;)"

"Just a part?!? ;) I have to admit that you are very intriguing and fu**g smart!!! Difficult to find... And I am also 100% sure you have other qualities, which I would love to know.... ;)"

"Straight back at ya ;) takes one to know one. It is my job, being a good mirror ;) I'm as curious as you, and perhaps I'd love to know stuff about you, you never thought to be of interest to me... BTW, is your business on Instagram?"

"Actually, I somehow think that we are very similar! (eyes wide) I like it (woot woot!)"

"Hmmm... in what way?"

"If you come to the Sky Bar, I'll tell you! ;) Nope, business not on Instagram. Personally, I don't even have it and I have someone taking care of the company's social networks but I'm not very happy about it."

"Awwww... love your effort! :) Instagram is important, let me know if you need support with this. In any case, set an account up for yourself. It's quite fun!"

"If you come to the Sky Bar we can talk about this! ;) LOL :-D :-D :-D"

"LOL :-D :-D :-D, you crack me up!"

"(Woot woot!) So, no way tonight? Come oooooonnnnnn!!!!!"

"I did say I was too much trouble ;)"

"OK... well, I will go back to my work and then maybe to the Sky Bar or to sleep! Thanks for the nice chat and thanks once more for the time you spent with me today! Sweet dreams! ;) XX"

"Sounds lovely, peaceful and productive. Have fun :) Pleasure is mine too."

But... I never heard from him since.

11 May, 2018

I have not seen Brigit in forever and I'm looking forward to seeing her again to catch up. She says she has news best shared in person. I reckon she's got a boyfriend. As our night call went on, she said,

"You know how you tell me to change what I say to myself? You have to do this now. You have to stop saying that you're too much trouble for men!"

It is true to some extent. I am too much trouble for many men. What I need and want combined is a big ask for the good men. Those who simply want to play, don't care. But a man who is looking for a life partner, who is thinking long term and marriage, will think seriously about the complications of being with a divorcee with a child. He will think about what he is signing up for and what the deal would entail with this 'package.' It is a big Ask, or perhaps, there just aren't many men capable of loving multi-dimensionally, and it isn't a criticism so much as a case of biology and pragmatism.

Self-love is tricky. Learning to say no, respecting my own time, honouring my space and truth, making myself a cup of cacao, treating myself to spa massages are starters. The real work is about reducing the buffer I put up, in order not to feel the darker emotions that arise from holding a toxic belief. And the only way to surface this belief is to increase my sensitivity to my inner guidance system. I walk the dark side to feel the dark feelings. What I mean by that is being able to tolerate those bad feelings, to feel judgment and to release judgment, to have clarity of discernment and choosing from a place of love.

Perhaps the truth to the matter is that there is an even deeper fear. You know how life is like an onion – you peel away one layer at a time, and sometimes you weep as a result.

A lot of the things I used to fear no longer have the same stronghold on me. I am able to dance with much of what life presents. I am a lot less attached now, a lot less needy, a lot more in flow and free. Having said that, I feel a lot more too, so it is much easier for me to drop deep within and feel my darkest most vulnerable spots, such as self-doubt, worries, and disappointments.

I don't think I realised how much my sex problems with Brendon had impacted me, in many different ways, good and bad. I feel both more *and* less confident. I also feel more *and* less competent. Perhaps as they say, ignorance, to some extent, is bliss!

But as with anything I have experienced, I would rather brave it than to go in blind. I also think it depends on the dynamic. With every person, the dance is different. The subtleties of vulnerable feelings and hormones pumping through the mix with the lust and love that arises in attraction.

I'm still learning to weave the energies... the spirit's calling, the soul's mission, and the human condition when it comes to sex. My conversations with both genders in the various age groups seem to offer enough evidence for me to conclude that I hold rather non-judgmental and liberal views, while simultaneously valuing the essence of culture, convention, and tradition as I evolve. I would not have arrived at this place without having experienced what I did with Brendon, and all the inner work I have been actively looking at, for as long as I can remember.

Brigit dished up my own words of advice – stop reinforcing unhelpful beliefs. Stop making excuses for others.

11 June, 2018

Following my desire to dance has led me to a whole lot of adventure!

Kiki and I went to a networking event at a nearby bistro and bar, where we met two Lithuanian guys. We laughed so much from their fun-loving silliness! Because the place closed early, they suggested we went to another lounge bar with live music that stayed open for a couple more hours. So, we went along to check it out. As we were leaving, Kiki commented how beautiful the potted plant on the table was. The tall guy simply lifted the pot and put it in his bag, and then left with it, for Kiki!

The lounge bar did not have a dancefloor, so Kiki and I decided to leave and head to a club nearby that had been recommended by someone we met there and then, called The Pod.

The minute we arrived, we got a sense that the place was... let's just say, rather unconventional. First, we were vetted after standing in line for what seemed like forever. By vetted I mean we were eyed from top to toe and we were asked interview-like questions. It was jam-packed, but well-staffed to ensure some sort of order. There were many open pods and the largest one stood in the middle. It was sleek, transparent, and spun around.

The hostesses were welcoming and plenty of people with money were offering drinks; I say people with money because we discovered from a quick Google search whilst in the queue, that the smallest table reservation had a minimum spend of £2000. The only problem was, because it was jam-packed, the only way one could dance was on the podium.

Thankfully, Kiki is a sport and a gem of a friend. We dropped our blazers, lost our pencil skirts, used our scarves for skirts, and pulled our hair up genie-like. Kiki joined me at the podium to dance, and boy, did we have a blast! The funny thing was, people thought we worked there! We received so many compliments. Then the lead hostess passed by us and on a whim, I blurted out, "Are you hiring podium dancers?"

Much to our surprise, she said yes!

"How much would I make?"

She came close, put her hands alluringly around my neck to pull me close and whispered, "Four nights, with tips, £55k plus."

*****

I have not written much about my financial thoughts, partly because I do not spend much time worrying about finances, and I truly wanted to positively focus on wealth creation. However, watching my savings dwindle is testing my ability to stay centred and thrive despite not knowing how or when my financial situation will change.

I have wiped out more than £55k since my divorce. I could do with being on a payroll and it helps me establish footprint for credit. I don't have to pay rent upfront, etc. To be honest, all my efforts to get paid work have been futile. There have been too many permutations.

How could I keep being a podium dancer under wraps? What happens if I meet my business clients or old colleagues? What would people say? Most of all, how would Yana be treated differently?

A lot of people believe podium dancers are sex workers. Imagine growing up being told that your mum is a whore! I don't think I can keep it quiet.

11 July, 2018

My opening night was stunning. I will always remember June 28, 2018. It was nerve-wrecking, yet the high dance vibes drowned out any nervous or anxious inner chatter that could have been a show stopper. With every move, I released old shit and began interacting with the room.

I cannot believe how swiftly the hiring process worked at The Pod. The entire assessment, induction, and improv choreography training took less than two weeks.

The best part is, I'm already clinking in the money box and I'm so relieved!

So far, I have not been spotted by anyone I know, I don't think. I am nervous about being recognised by someone at Yana's school, of course. But maybe this is my work. This is me. I make no apologies. There is no shame to my work. I am a professional dancer, albeit without ballet training, nor any dance qualification. The ironic thing is, no Pod customers have asked me to go home with them to date. Perhaps it's early days but I am surprised because almost every time I went dancing with the girls, men would have tried to take me home with them. It's so ironic.

I did meet a charming French chap yesterday. It was after work and I finished early. I was walking past Bar Vivva and bumped into Cath. So, I stopped to catch up when I accidentally kicked the pint glass on the floor towards this French chap. His group made such a fuss, and I tried to be playful but I was too tired. He came back to apologise on behalf of his friends and asked if he could get me coffee the next day.

I have developed a few strategic self-selection lines that help me vet men upfront. One of these is to state that I have a child. Once, I was at a very posh bar, getting myself a drink, when a very handsome British man of mixed parentage said, 'Fancy having an old-fashioned?'

We exchanged pleasantries, and as I mentioned my daughter, he practically disappeared with his friends, leaving one behind to talk to me. He re-emerged after an hour or so, to get his friend, and said to me, 'You look after yourself, ok,' and then left. I believe he is also more than a decade younger. Generous perhaps, but... nay.

Speaking of generous, once a man started talking to me at the buffet table, knowing I was with Yana. He paid me several compliments, mentioned he also has a daughter, and he looked like he was going to ask for my number. I cut the conversation short each time he tried to open one. For some reason, I did not think he was 'my type,' even though, ask me to describe 'my type,' and I will tell you, 'I can't!' You know what? He paid for my lunch with Yana that day. When I asked for the bill, the waiter told me, 'the guy who was sitting over there (now empty table) has paid for you.' I was touched by his gesture. It challenged my paradigm. I always believed that guys have an ulterior motive when they bought me stuff.

Oh, back to the French chap. I said to him, 'I'm taking my daughter out, and being a working single mum, time with her is so precious.' He said, 'When would be good then?'

Interesting line, I thought to myself. Perhaps he has kids, too. Usually the reaction I get would be, 'Oh, how old is she?' And they usually drop the asking or ask me to call them instead.

I'm seeing the French chap in a couple of days.

Separately, Kiki said I ought to shift paradigms, tell my story as podium dancer, and clear the stigma associated with night club dancing. More than that, I never knew there would be so many mothers who work in night clubs because the hours work for them as primary carers. Many are slightly ashamed because 'good mums' stay out of night clubs, and 'good mums' are not single mums working in night clubs. 'She probably got pregnant by some random guy in this club,' was a comment overheard by one of my colleagues about her. How sad.

11 August, 2018

It's a little over a month. I have received not only pay checks but many party and meal invitations, and absolutely no requests for sexual services. Can you believe it?

I'm not sure whether this is a good sign or a bad sign!

Perhaps I am not sexy enough, just entertaining enough!

Whatever it is, it is good for me. I do think it's just a matter of time though. Nevertheless, I am taking extra work and I have developed a fan base for my stage name. Yana has met my colleagues at picnics, afternoon tea, and she has seen photos of my performances and even witnessed me live on stage, when the environment is more family-friendly.

I have met many people. Some love the night scene that consists of booze and sex, while some are into letting hair down in a space where the "dark side" can come out and play. The old me would have viewed these people as superficial, material, shallow, low vibe folks who do not know true peace and happiness. Now that I am walking in their shoes, I can say that we are responsible for creating that sense of separation.

The creative aspect, the hearts and minds, are all being tuned by the unique journey each of us are on. The amount of laughter that goes on in the room, the amount of physical movement, alcohol notwithstanding, there comes a moment when time literally expands and the cacophony melds into one singular tone of humanity that is very silent.

I have had the most fun-filled conversations that are nothing but superficial, because all you need is a moment, a window, to have a snapshot into people's souls, hearts, and truth.

With the improv choreography concept, no two evenings are ever the same, and my creativity has been expanding from purely mind sourced to engage and co-create with a live audience. Perhaps it is how my fans perceive me. I come across as someone who is very receptive and non-judgmental towards what people tell me, and my being vulnerable somehow makes me someone the audience knows intimately, despite being an entertainer at arm's length. Somehow, I have become someone strangers feel comfortable sharing their best kept secrets with.

While I enjoy dancing, a perk that I absolutely love is the party conversations I am privy to. I get a kick out of surprising guests and my clients with my anecdotes from my past work experience because most people assume I am a performing artist and an accidental social escort, or as some establishments call it, a Public Relations Officer. I have yet to meet anyone who believes me when I tell them my age and that I am divorced with a child. Mostly they think I am a fresh graduate starting out. Perhaps against this backdrop of assumption, I come across as particularly impressive!

I seem to still be attracting younger men, which is annoying because they are serious time wasters. While the younger men are bolder, braver, more engaging and spontaneous than the older men, the older men are more reliable, thoughtful, generous and focused. Of course, I'm broad brushing. In any case, I don't suppose I'm clear with regards to finding a partner, and maybe this is why.

I've started a side hobby of helping girlfriends increase the attraction factor and helping guy friends get the girl. The twist to this hobby is the intimacy aspect for couples – learning to be so self-responsible for one's own intimate pleasure and comfortable in one's own skin, that it allows freedom of expression, within educated boundaries, to be playful with each other in an intimate private relationship. What was once so taboo to even talk about in my traditional upbringing, what once made me blush or cringe, now doesn't bother me in the slightest.

There is one thing that I still do not do... sex-ting.

With the younger men, many go down that route, perhaps as a way to wank off. I have received photos of dicks, as if the photos did anything for me. I receive booty calls from people I have never slept with. Flirtation, erotica exchanges, and fantasy conversations are entertaining, but totally distracting. Once, I was out having dinner with a potential boyfriend and my phone flashed with messages like, "When are you coming for cuddles?" "I want to lick your pussy." "I can give you a massage." "Come stay at mine tomorrow." Eventually I switched it off!

Oh, and I had an interesting twist to sex-ting with the French chap, whose name is Francois. After that one meeting we had, we began exchanging seductive, playful, romantic texts... and we met up another time, by chance, and he stole more kisses and began getting dates in the diary for going out and hanging out at each other's homes.

As if by Divine intervention, however, I fell ill, and both

impromptu and planned meet-ups never took place for a month. Soon, the 'full day trip' we had planned drew near. As the saying goes, "Time tells." I came across a quote once – 'If the words don't add up, it's usually because the truth wasn't included in the equation.'

So, our text exchanges had been rather fun and engaging... but after a while, I felt it to be more about luring me into 'his den' rather than finding opportunities to grab a coffee or asking me things to get to know me as a person. He would be full-on for a few days, then disappear without a word... and return like this:

"Hiya, how was London without me?"

With greater clarity about what I want, not just from this particular encounter, but from my experience post-divorce, and hopefully, more non-attachment, elegance and pure joy, I engaged:

"How was Dubrovnik without me?"

"Not bad at all despite you not being here. Speaking of holidays, are we still off next week?"

"I'm a bit confused... I think I asked some time ago about next week but you were silent so I thought you lost interest. I really like you. We've got chemistry. But you swing hot and cold, so I don't know how to place you. I don't feel you are invested in getting to know me as a person. I sense some confusion as to what you want. So I'm going to take some space too, cos I don't want to get closer to someone whose not sure/clear about what he wants."

"I'm sorry, what? Last time we spoke about it, we agreed to do a day trip. So what happened?"

"Did we? Maybe I missed it. Sorry."

"I mean in my mind, it was clear it was happening. But now you said you want some space?"

"Yeah, I don't do well at hook ups or Friends with Benefits... it started to feel like it was heading that way. I'm a bit tired and could do with some consistency in my life. I didn't know it was happening, to be honest, cos I got no clear answer. Think you were more into the sleepover before and after the day trip, but I could be wrong. I'm cool though. I hold you in equal esteem."

"When did you ask? I'm really surprised by this, I was convinced it was happening. But anyway, we didn't really discuss it. So I guess better sooner than later."

Two hours later...

"So do you know what you want?"

"I do."

Fourteen hours later...

"And what is it?"

"A relationship... An open, honest, trusting, meaningful connection, in a mutually rewarding, deeply valued one."

Six hours later...

"Sounds wonderful. I really hope you'll find it. As you said, I'm not sure I can give you that."

"Thank you :)"

Thirty-six hours later...

"So, do you still wanna see me?"

"No. Of course, I don't mind when we hang out with friends."

"As friends or with friends?"

"Both. You're fun to hang out with."

"And so are you. Will be hard not to kiss you though."

"Easy, just think of the cost and you'll figure that it's too much to cross the line."

"Oh really? What cost :)?"

I left it, and he has never texted again since.

The end of Francois.

That aside, the private moments I shared with both male and female clients I met at work, all without sexual intercourse, got me to a place of realisation that ultimately, everyone wants to feel safe, everyone has some shame and guilt, and everyone deserves to receive and give pleasure. Parents have started to confide in me, not just about their marital sex, but about the rites of passage for their children. I have started to charge a fee purely for the fact that I started to talk to people I do not even know and rewarding my friends for their referral.

I guess part of the appeal is that I am not too 'out there in the woods,' nor am I too 'clinical and academic.' I am a mom who grew from humble beginnings in a conservative family, as an innocent, tradition-bound girl who has seen the world and walked the footsteps of people from all walks of life, to be a "street-wise spirit, self-aware, truthful and genuine," who bridges the duality in the matrix, to hold space as everyone expands.

'The new Woman of Light,' as described by one of my fans.

'Not a prostitute nor a temple priestess, not a Goddess

nor a Shaman gone wrong. Not a surrogate nor a 'Firewomen' type sex educator. Not a psychotherapist nor a sexologist. Not a coach nor a social escort, not a Tarot card reader nor Reiki healer. But each are in her as she speaks your unique guidance and guides you to listen to your own greatest teacher and creator,' said another.

For me, I am a woman, being whole. Neither of light nor of dark, but of One.

11 September, 2018

Oh my gosh! I can hardly contain my excitement! I'm super thrilled I could break this laptop typing! The office of Matt Huxley, the world's most famous dating and relationship coach, left me a voice message today. They said they love my ideas and have a project they want to discuss with me. I also read the emails that followed and we have scheduled a call to connect and iron out the details. If all goes well, I'm set to go to LA for a couple of weeks.

I can hardly breathe... it's like a dream come true. Something good could come out of all my adventure, it seems! Of course, I am thrilled that they took a serious look at my profile and proposal and are open to co-creating something new with me.

A few weeks ago, it seemed as if my life had turned upside down. A video of me at work, edited to look way bad, went viral with my real name plastered everywhere. I was so worried about Yana.

My real girlfriends were fine and totally supportive. My family was also cool. But the guys I was dating... that was a different story. The Brazilian chap was the coolest about it, maybe because he has known me the longest. The Turkish guy, on the other hand, started to step up his game in the wrong way; I'm not sure what he is thinking. The Italian one got pissed off, saying we had a weird destiny, and that he could have rescued me from all this shame but because I did not like him enough in that way, I ended up harming myself?

Gosh – the stuff that goes on in people's heads, one can only wonder...

I mentioned the video to Huxley's team, just to pre-empt. It turns out they knew already, and do not see how this would negatively impact our collaboration.

11 October, 2018

Things with Huxley's team got off to the right start. And as I process what's been going on, how my life has changed so much in the last couple of years, I entered the process of merging, of becoming one, of bridging the divide. What I mean by this is the two worlds that I walk – conveniently labelled as Spiritual and Material– have been melding naturally... magical alchemy, in beauty. While I can understand the labels and what they mean, and the groups that sit in each of the categories, the descriptors and differentiation no longer hold much substance for me.

I discovered that my proposal got onto Huxley's radar because someone in his team is a fan of The Pod, and apparently, I have met him, but they have been instructed to keep his identity a secret until I go to LA. Apparently, even my arrival into the office is in scope for filming.

I am discovering how much of a spiritual snob I have been. Perhaps different adventure draws out different aspects of me.

Examining how my life looks today, based on my past beliefs, there is nothing spiritual about it; nothing I would regard as spiritual anyway. Yet, I feel good. Centred. Happy. My basic needs are met.

I am not on any 'save the world' missions. Perhaps, for as long as I can remember, this is the first time I felt that my 'superficial entertainment work' is good enough... that

I am good enough.

My work sits in the world.

There's no point colluding in the spiritual circle to perpetuate anger towards those deemed unloving, selfish and desirous, and hurl covert judgments or avoid life and living altogether. There's no point colluding in the 'normal world' (I use 'normal' because a fellow spiritual sibling who identifies with the Angel energy of Metatron once said to me that he cannot be with a 'normal' woman anymore) to perpetuate anger towards those deemed as up in the clouds, having God complex and not contributing to the world in any real way.

I think I'm coming to a point where I prefer to believe in the best for every situation rather than the need to be right. Life is so full of surprises. And I am grateful to all my supporters.

A year ago, I would never have thought the Divine Masculine would show up in this way, in the darkness. The embodiment surprised me. It all started about a year ago when my finances went pear-shaped, and after I just got that news from my broker that my refinancing fell through, I went for drinks with Jason. I felt my tears welling up, and he immediately took my hand, looked me in the eye and said, "Don't worry, we'll take care of you," seeming to know who he was referring to when he said 'we.'

Fast-forward a year and I do feel the collective 'we' as the masculine energy that provides the structure so the feminine energy can just be and create...but not in the way I imagined.

Jason began for me, as a way for men (and some women)

who channels the masculine energy in form of money passing through them as the super conductor of energy. He said to me, 'If I were to enjoy your company and bought you coffee at least once a week, that would be roughly £20 per month. If you have one hundred people who believe in you, invested in keeping you well, and want to see you live your best life because it feeds the world, then you will receive £2000 every month, to do what you do best – being with people.'

He prototyped this for me by getting five others in his circle who knew me well enough, to commit to what he committed for me. His parting words were:

"Never underestimate your power, and never undervalue your gifts, especially the powerful gift of your presence."

I am so grateful to have so many providers. Sometimes I catch myself feeling undeserving... like my life, my work, my being, is not worth people spending £20 every month... because I'm not serving any Divine mission, not saving lives or alleviating hunger. Most of all, because I'm having fun. It flushes out this internalised belief I uncovered that in order for me to deserve gifts, I must work hard and not have fun. I don't feel like I deserved to receive other people's earned money to have fun.

11 November, 2018

Today is a momentous day.

I have finally calmed down slightly. It is all surreal. I cannot believe it... yet.

I felt it coming last night. I looked in the night sky and the slither of moon left me feeling like the Sky Angel was smiling down upon me. I smiled back and said hello, and as I connected with my heart towards the crescent, I moved to dance.

It was most delightful! The slow unfolding of each movement allowed my body to stretch in opposite directions in a fluid way to take in all the messages and love moving through my surroundings. As my fingers each opened up and curved back in, every joint doing mini-twirls, there was a pause where my head was drawn to the earth, my feet launching up like rockets.

This morning, I woke up after a deep sleep to move swiftly in my dreamy state to brush my teeth. As I opened my eyes, instead of commenting how groggy, puffy, wrinkly, or horrible I looked, I laughed at myself because a funny thought came to mind. I looked like I just made love to the Sky Angel! I found myself feeling rather sexy but oddly, looking the total opposite of what I would describe as sexy.

Morning cuppa in hand, I went to my inbox and I saw the email from Oprah's team. My heart sank momentarily because I believed that if it was good news, it would have been a phone call instead of an email. So, I took a deep breath and scanned the note.

I did a double take when I realised it was good news!

The network wants me to do a few things:

- write and direct a fun feature for a women's campaign
- be interviewed and perform my signature dance live
- be filmed for promos

OMG!

And wait, wait... guess what the timestamp of the email was?

11:11

Perhaps if I didn't have such a happy hippie vibe with 11:11, I would have gotten worried and spooked out. But I took it as a positive sign that this new beginning marks the end of a whole era... fully satisfied as I am with my life post-divorce as a sexologist's ex-wife, it is time for me to move on.

Next Saturday, I will be going for yoga, massage and a spa day, followed by warming hug-in-a -mug kind of cacao cocktails in the evening at The Better Tail, then finish with some dipping at The Vondue... with none other than my BFFs Kiki, Brigit, Evelyn, Inez, and Diane. We will be dreaming up how we want to be feeling when we next get together, across the pond, on set.

Yes, I get to bring them with me to LA for the project with Matt Huxley!

I still can't believe it.

11 November, 2020

It's 1:11 in the morning, and I am writing with Emilio's music playing in the background, under the stars. This is a dream come true. I have always wanted to be under the stars. Yesterday, I was writing exactly that on my Instagram, and as I typed the word Star, Yana came to me with Cloudbabies on the iPad, showing me the part where the babies were stringing stars and she said she wanted to do that too. The serendipity was enchanting, and it is carrying through to me now as if by magic, because I am looking up and I see a line of stars as if one of the Cloudbabies was stringing them for me, just like how I am stringing these alphabets and words.

Vince walks to Kerry, hugs her tight, gives her a kiss, and says, "Stay up as late as you want Starlight Owl, I'll be dreaming of you!"

Kerry replies, "I love you!"

God, I love that man.

How things change in just a few years. I never thought I would end up sharing a life with someone like him. Vince is a total game changer.

It has often been said that people are not perfect and therein lies the perfection in God's design. As I look at him, and as I experience how we share our lives with each other, I realise that there are perfect moments, where everything seems to slide in place. With Vince, I discovered that we share so much more of in-sync communication, beyond words, beyond time, beyond space. The energy is easy flowing. No push and pull from the solar plexus, only push and pull from the sacral, and sometimes a stand-off followed by an easing of that for flow to resume.

It's the powerful moments that make us return to each other every day, to want to be with each other, to play and have fun, to feel safe yet passionate at the same time. He has done practically zero training in psychology or sexology, or any of those softer humanistic fields. He works the land, listens with his body, and does with his mind.

When we laugh, sometimes it can get so crazy and deep that we just want to jump on each other like playmates with adult privileges. We know attraction, we understand the mechanics of it, we talk about stuff that is important for us, we cut the noise out and stay in alignment with each of our own greatest glorious selves. This is our biggest blessing, our priceless gift, for ourselves and for each other.

When sharing, we come from a heart space that is free from personal agendas and is taken in from that same trusting open place. The intimacy is electrifying. The safe space transforms to a desirous sacred bubble for two that feels like home.

Perhaps it is timing, perhaps it is Divine... who knows why we are a couple?

Vince works in agriculture and construction. We met at a gay bar.

Vince loves spoiling me with the mundane, i.e. forget fancy gifts, he shares his life with me in every way, such that his wealth is insignificant next to the thing he shares.

Vince is not a fan of getting high nor drunk.

Vince is unafraid of anything I share with him, including my mood swings.

Vince trusts me completely, and he believes in me, no if's and but's.

Vince cracks me up. He knows when I need my quiet time. He knows when I just need to talk. He knows the best cure for my emotional ailments is cuddles.

Vince has no qualms experimenting with me in our sexual space. We both run high with passion and sacred lust!

Vince adores Yana and whether he has his 'own' biological child or not with me is unimportant to him, because in his words, 'I'm marrying you to be with you, to serve, honour and cherish you as the love of my human life. I'm marrying you because I want to create that safe cocoon with you, and to celebrate our union in the best way I know how to – with all of me. I'm a traditional old soul and the luckiest man to find another traditional old soul.'

I never cried so much and laughed so much in one evening, the night he proposed.

Vince and I have an open relationship. Our definition of open relationship is to be open and honest with each other about anything that is important to each of us, including our sacred sexual intimacy space, especially if we choose to introduce other elements, including people, into it. There is to be no deception. It seems as if we are monogamous in an open and conscious way.

We maintain our rights to privacy, and by that, we can be selective about the thoughts and opinions we share with each other, but in terms of feelings we commit to being totally transparent and self-responsible.

And as I gaze at this responsibly sourced giant green diamond ring under the stars, sitting above the gold wedding band, I wonder... while I believed that all that glitters are not gold, and diamonds aren't truly a girl's best friend, and that these material things are not important to me, I was pushed by forces beyond me to raise my game and not fall into judgement for how he ought to be spending his time, energy and money, and instead, receive all these material blessings believing that I truly deserve without feeling guilty or shameful. That spiritual snob side of me has dropped her judgment on desire and financial wealth.

I have been able to share my wealth in ways I previously only dreamed of. I have opened up the space for new products and new businesses to be birthed. I have enjoyed hosting friends and their friends at home and connected people who have done amazing things together.

There was one BIG stubborn old belief that I had to face, that scratches at me like a horrible ghoulish cat. Every day that I have been with him, I have been chipping away at this belief, cleansing my pride and my ego as a process, some would describe.

The belief…

Saying yes to a relationship with him, meant going out to the world with the label 'gold-digging cougar' on my forehead. Literally.

Why?

Because Vince is 12 years younger than me, with a physique and wallet the envy of many.

And guess what he said when he first learnt about my age, my marital status, and my job?

'Does it matter?'

And guess what we did right after that scary conversation?

Danced, sang, and laughed all night through to the break of dawn.

Somewhere in there, my insecurities and self-doubt reared its head, several times. I was doubtful that he could see beyond my human body, that once we get into the routine, the age gap would pose an issue. Why would he bother to get married at all when he can keep doing what he's been doing, freely? I guess I was worried and hopeful, but most of all, I was buffering fear and pain. Putting it in perspective, the ultimate fears of all fears, masked by many logical reasons or rationale, is the fear of death... the fear of what we do not know, and what we have projected as the worst possible outcome.

But it was these words that allowed me to hold strong while moving forward with courage:

'Kerry, I see you. Your soul, your spirit, whatever that spunk is, you dance in my heart. And that's what matters to me. We are both crazy, but we are cool, so let's do crazy cool together!'

I can hear my shadow speaking, 'There you go again, you sucker of romance, you never learn. He's going to break your heart again, the way all the rest have done before him. You've had your fun, so let it go and cut your losses because you're safer without him.'

Very brutal this self-doubt.

My antidote?

I drew this shadow, laughed at myself being rubbish at drawing, then went for Zumba and comedy club. In the past, I would have judged this as avoidance. But you know what? I no longer feel this way. Perhaps it was a process I had to go through to come to a particular awareness, but is awareness necessary at all? I wonder.

Then I hear Vince's voice:

'Does it matter?'

Haha. I have a new 'allowing-mation': Laugh, dance and have fun.

I allow myself Play... to engage in playfulness with sheer joy and freedom!

www.ingramcontent.com/pod-product-compliance
Lightning Source LLC
Chambersburg PA
CBHW030642190726
48286CB00008B/2623

* 9 7 8 1 9 1 3 0 3 6 3 6 2 *